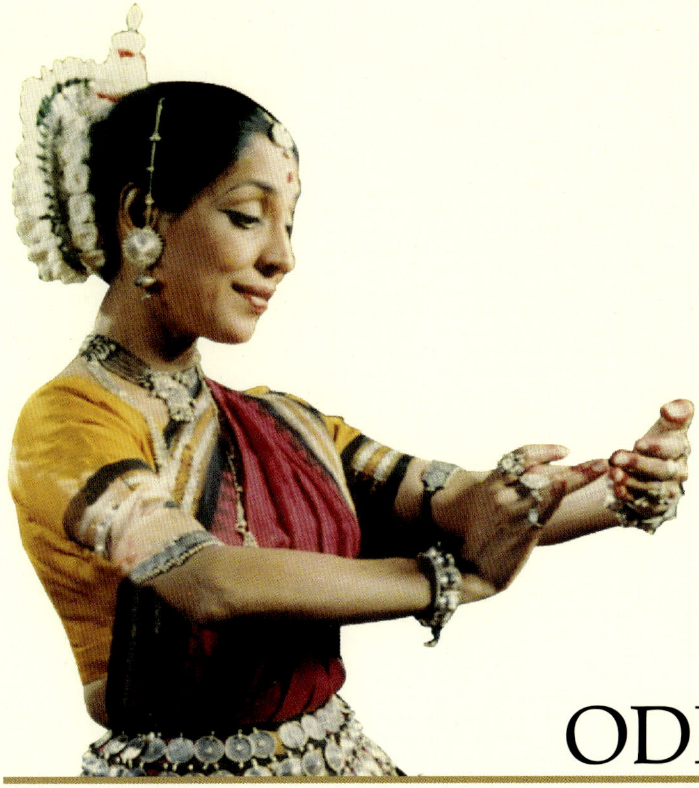

ODISSI

AN INDIAN CLASSICAL DANCE FORM

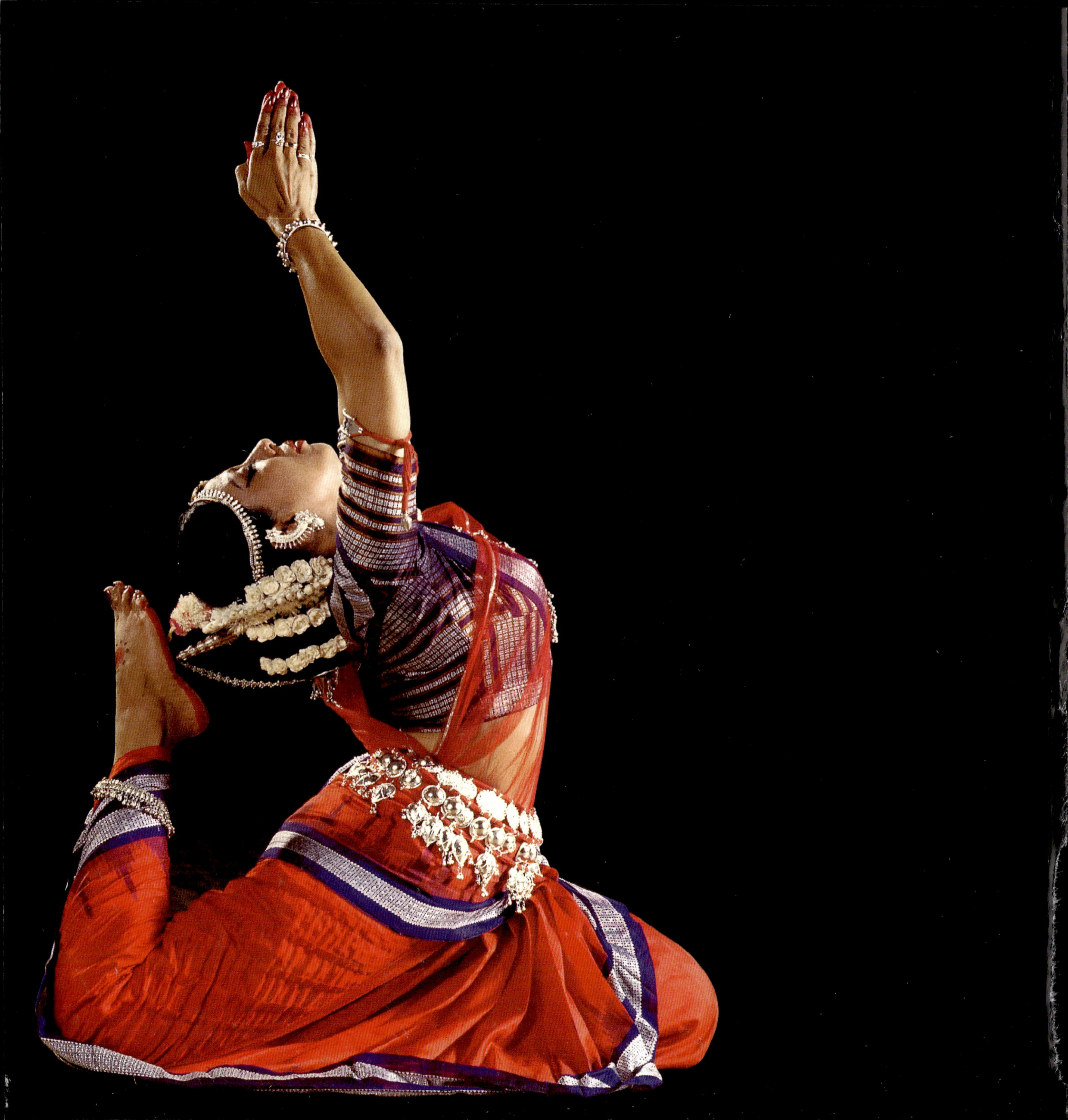

Priyambada Mohanty Hejmadi
Ahalya Hejmadi Patnaik

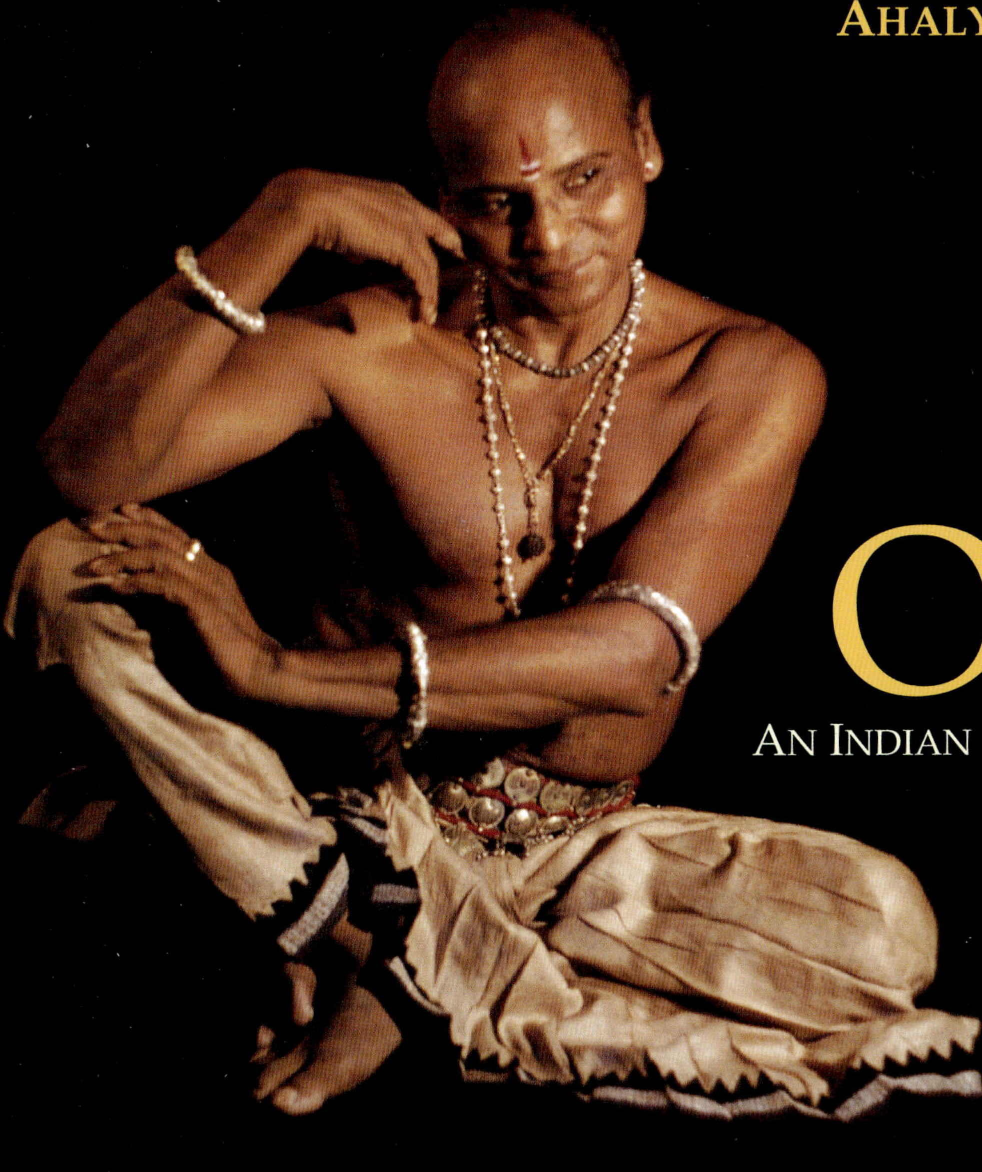

Odissi

An Indian Classical Dance Form

Aryan Books International
New Delhi

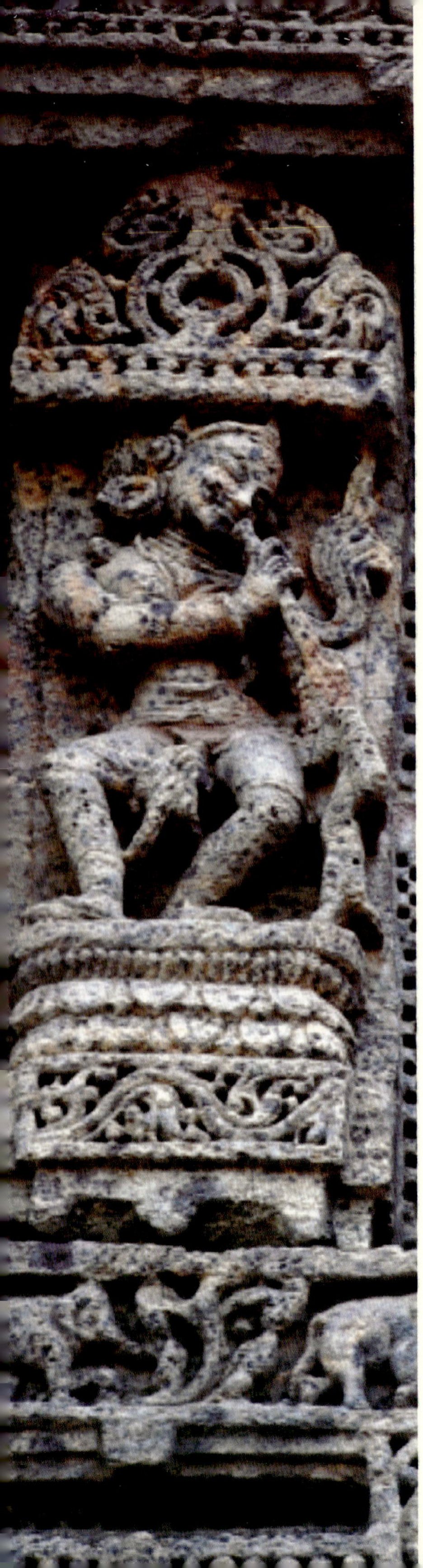

ODISSI
An Indian Classical Dance Form

ISBN-81-7305-324-3

Photo credits:
Sangeet Natak Akademi; Avinash Pasricha-page i, ii, vi, x, xii, 89, 117;
Sonal Mansingh-vi, 117; Ratikanta Mahapatra-x, 89;
Madhavi Mudgal-i; Aruna Mohanty-105;
Sadasiba Pradhan-10, 11; Rabinarayan Panda-46.

Published in **2007** by :
ARYAN BOOKS INTERNATIONAL
Pooja Apartments, 4B, Ansari Road, Darya Ganj, New Delhi-110 002 (India)
Tel.: 23287589, 23255799; Fax: 91-11-23270385
E-mail: aryanbooks@vsnl.com

Design: Kamal Purna Jammual
Computer Typeset and Printed in India at
ABI Prints & Publishing Co., New Delhi

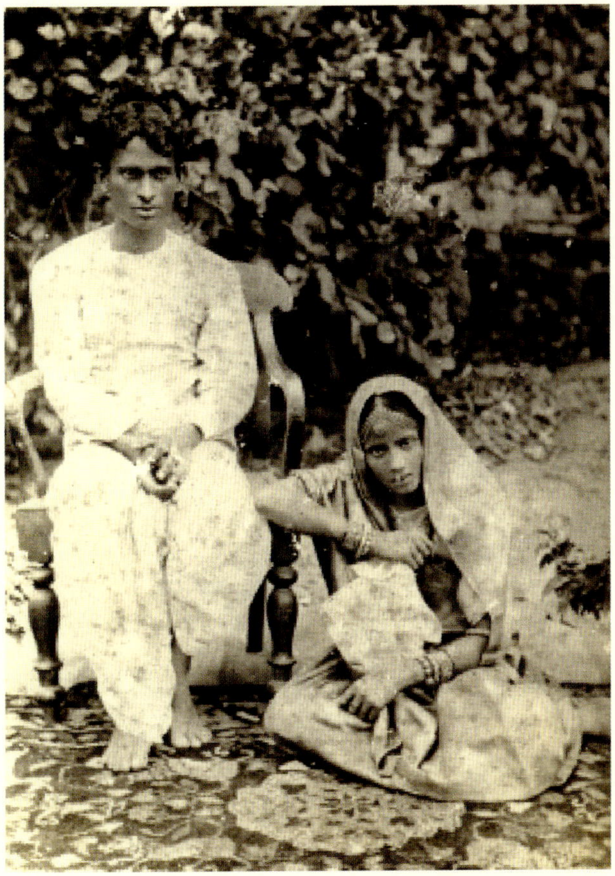

This book is dedicated to the memories of

Shri Bhagabat Charan Mohanty and Shrimati Nisamoni Devi, for opening the window

to the beautiful world of art and culture for their daughter Priyambada and granddaughter Ahalya

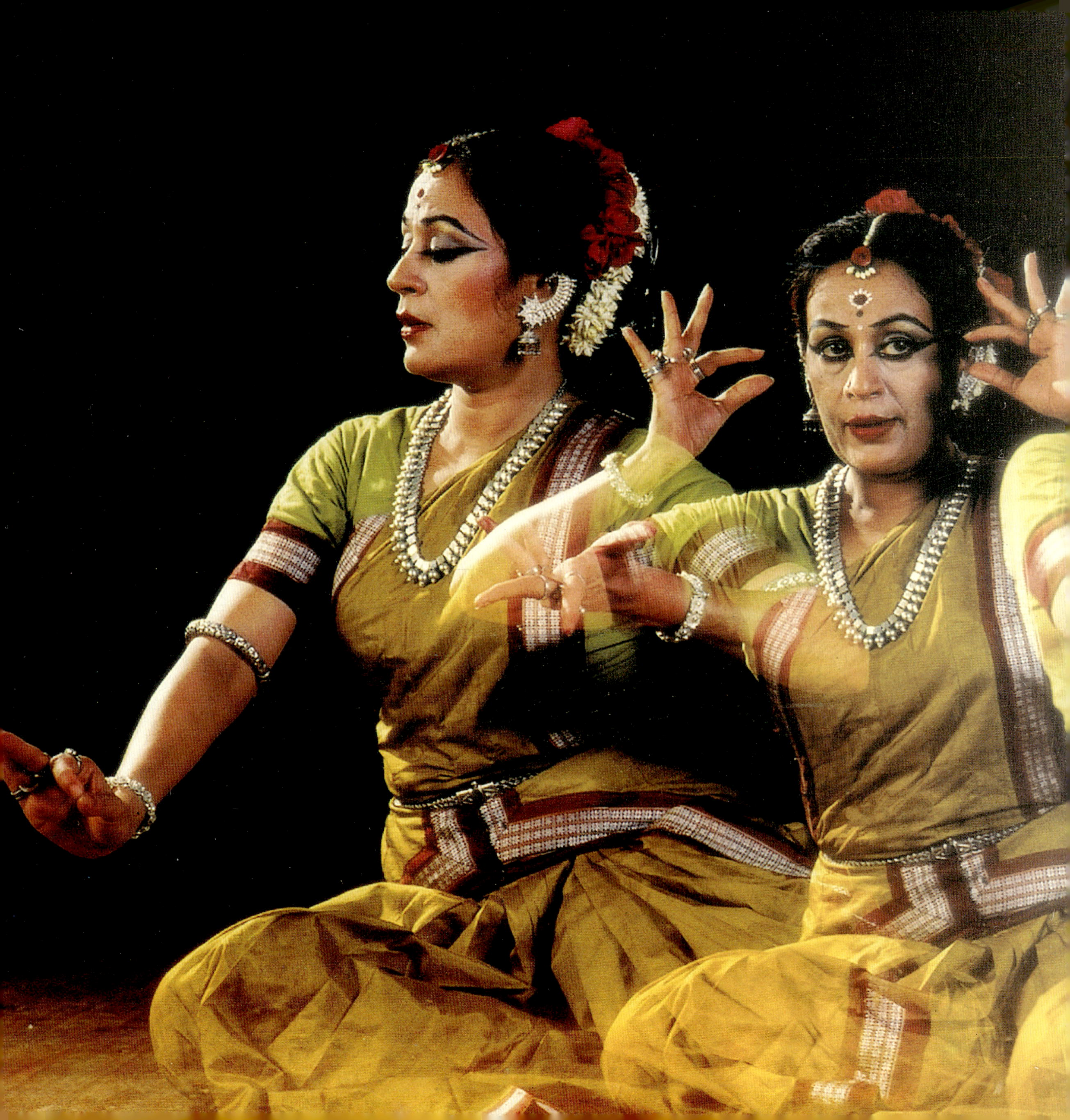

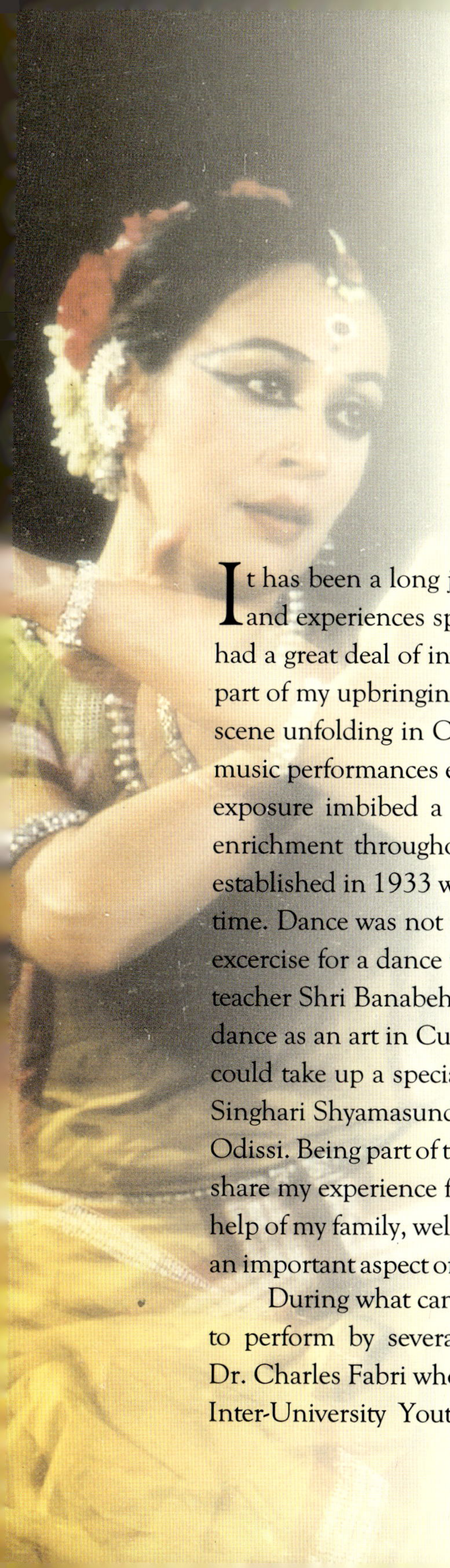

PREFACE

It has been a long journey to publish this book covering events, happenings and experiences spanning over almost 60 years. Being born to a family who had a great deal of involvement in art and culture, I learnt music and dance as part of my upbringing. Since, my parents were actively involved in the cultural scene unfolding in Cuttack in 1940's, I had the opportunity to attend theatre, music performances even before I understood what they meant. But, slowly the exposure imbibed a cultural temper which has been of enormous personal enrichment throughout my life. I learnt music in the Utkal Sangeet Samaj established in 1933 which was the centre for all the practicing musicians of the time. Dance was not taught those days, but happened to me as a rehabilitation excercise for a dance teacher arriving in Cuttack to make a living. I can say the teacher Shri Banabehari Maity became very much a part of the development of dance as an art in Cuttack. Having mastered the footwork under his training, I could take up a special dance which was taught by the Doyen of Odissi music Singhari Shyamasunder Kar. This dance manifested itself into the modern day Odissi. Being part of the process I thought that it will be proper to document and share my experience for posterity. Actually, it has been the encouragement and help of my family, well wishers and friends that I have put together what I feel is an important aspect of the emergence of Odissi.

During what can be referred to as the struggling period, I was encouraged to perform by several eminent people who are no more. I am grateful to Dr. Charles Fabri whose generous comments in 1954, on my dance at the First Inter-University Youth Festival was so critical for the revival of Odissi. He encouraged me to take it up and arranged the full evening programme in Sapru House and invited Madam Indira Gandhi to see the new form of dance. His association with Dr. Mayadhar Mansingh, the well known poet from Orissa led the latter to take a keen interest in the endeavour. Dr. Mansingh was a contemporary and friend of my father, and took personal interest in my dance and Odissi as a whole. I remember him coming to our house, supervising the compositions with the help of Pandit Banambar Acharya for *Geeta Govinda astapadis*. Dr. Mansingh was keen that everyone should understand the lyrics used and translated many songs into English which I have included in this book.

It was the generosity of many well wishers that I could collect some rare materials. I express my gratitude to poet and littérateur Dr. J.P. Das for providing me with copies of Record of Rights, rare articles and other documents related to *mahari seva* in the Jagannath Temple. My friend Shyamali Bardhan has been a source of strength from accompanying me to Delhi for the first ever full evening performance in New Delhi in 1961 to providing me with a copy of the rare article on *maharis* dated 1912; my special thanks to her.

The nomenclature of *mahari* has been of interest and my thanks to Professor K.S. Behera for sharing his thoughts and providing me with important documents. It was not easy to get a drawing of the *Kandarpa Ratha* from the Jagannath Temple. I thank Dedadutta Samantasinghar for his help. Thanks are due to Shri Ramahari Das for providing important information on Odissi music.

This book would not have seen the day without the constant encouragement of my family specially my sister Shrimati Annapurna Devi and brother Shri Prakash Chandra Mohanty. I feel privileged to have them as my siblings. It is for the record that Ahalya, my co-author generously decided that I should write the preface on our behalf. I am grateful to Dr. Sadasiba Pradhan for his help in the preparation of the index, bibliography and other help in publication. Last but not the least, a special thanks to Mr. Vikas Arya of Aryan Books International, for his personal interest in publishing the book.

Priyambada Mohanty Hejmadi

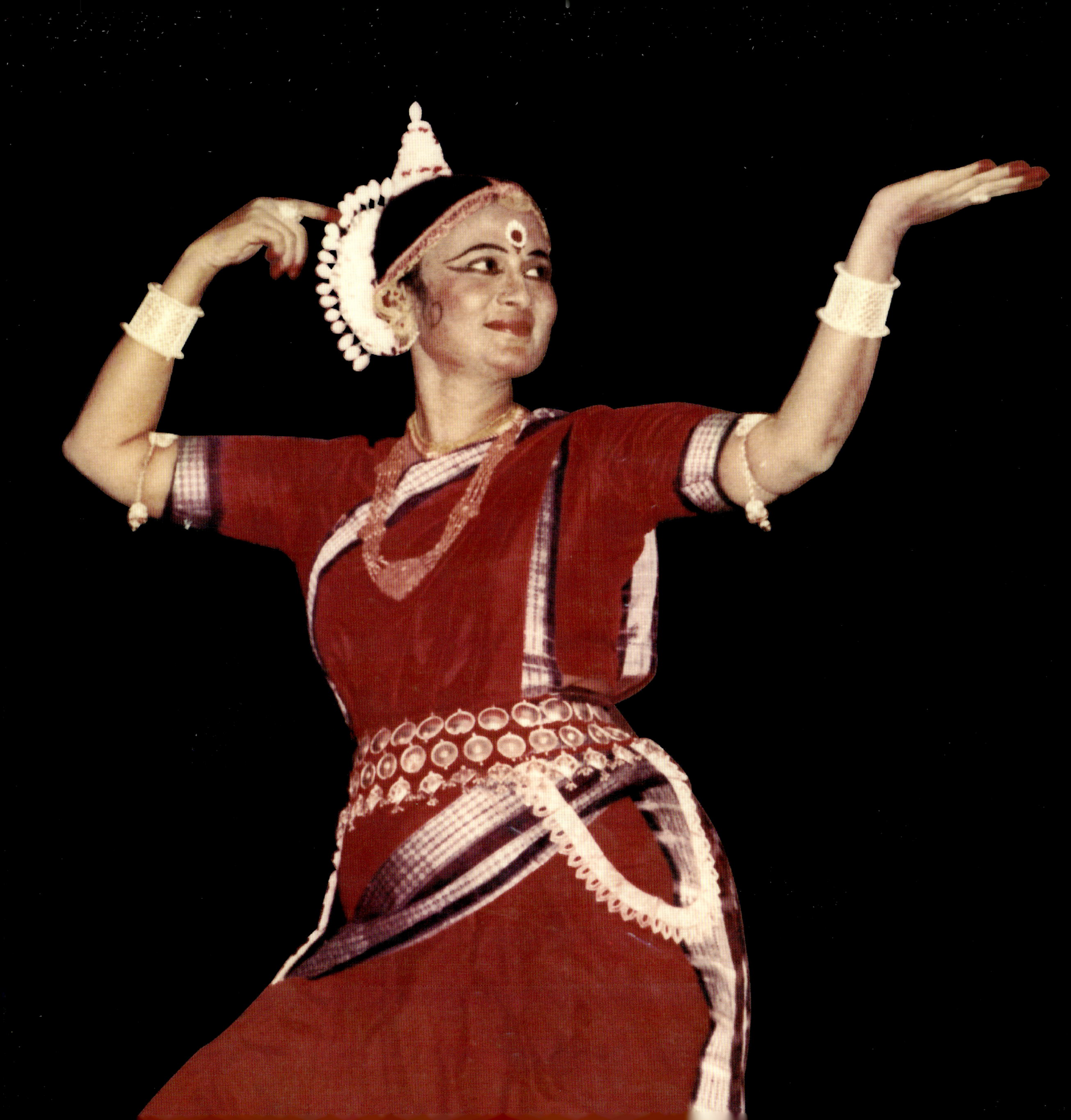

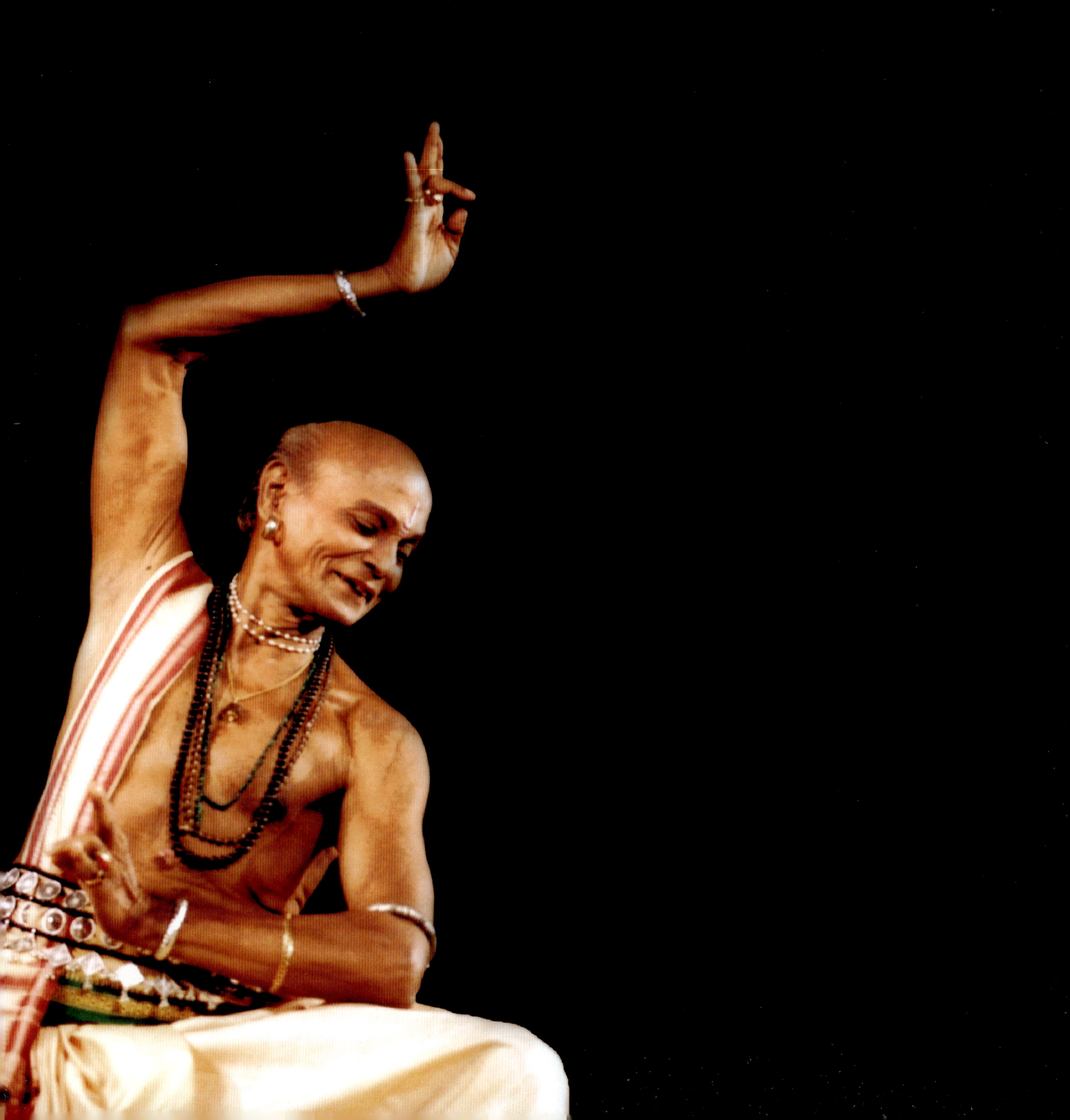

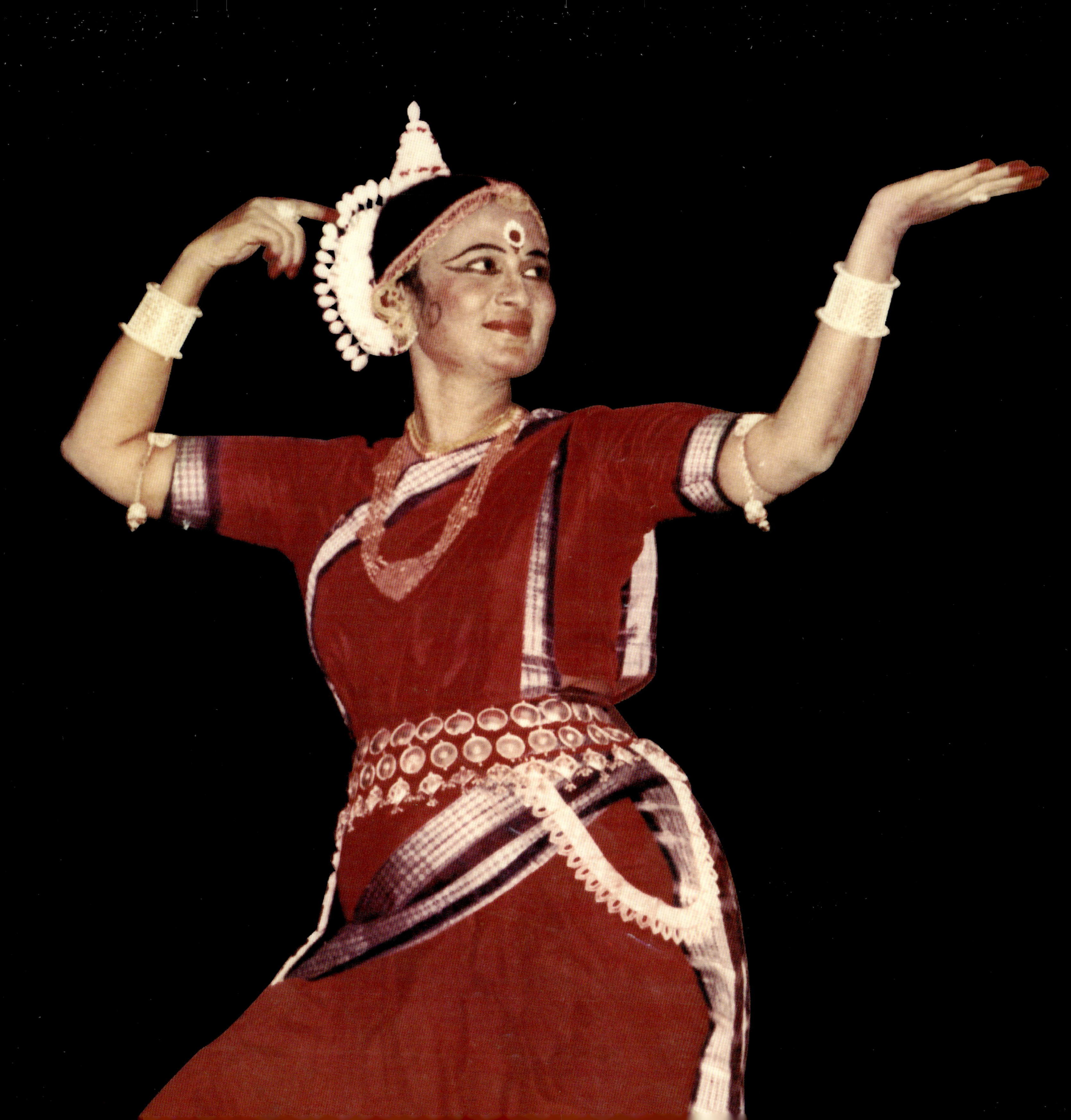

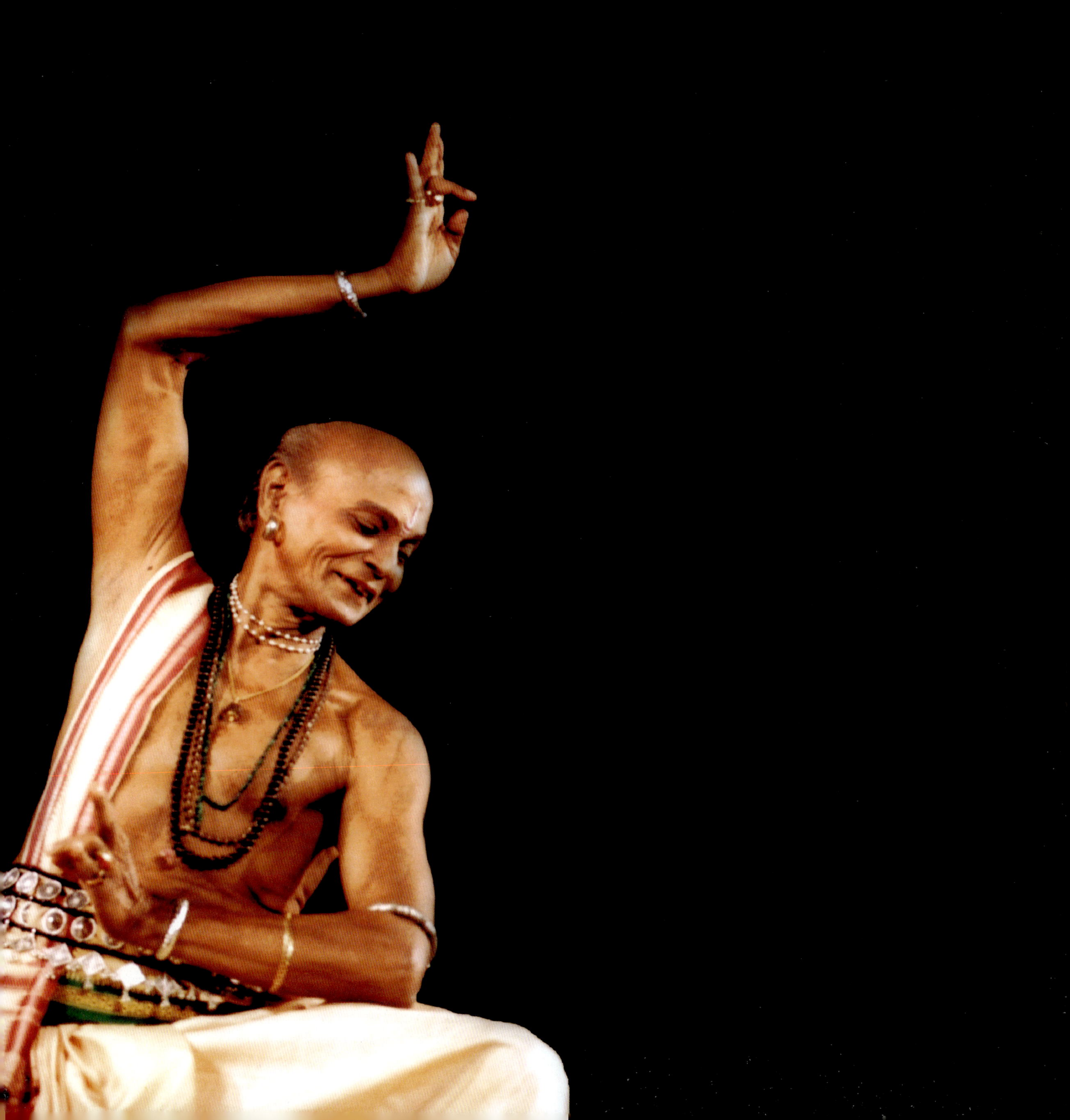

CONTENTS

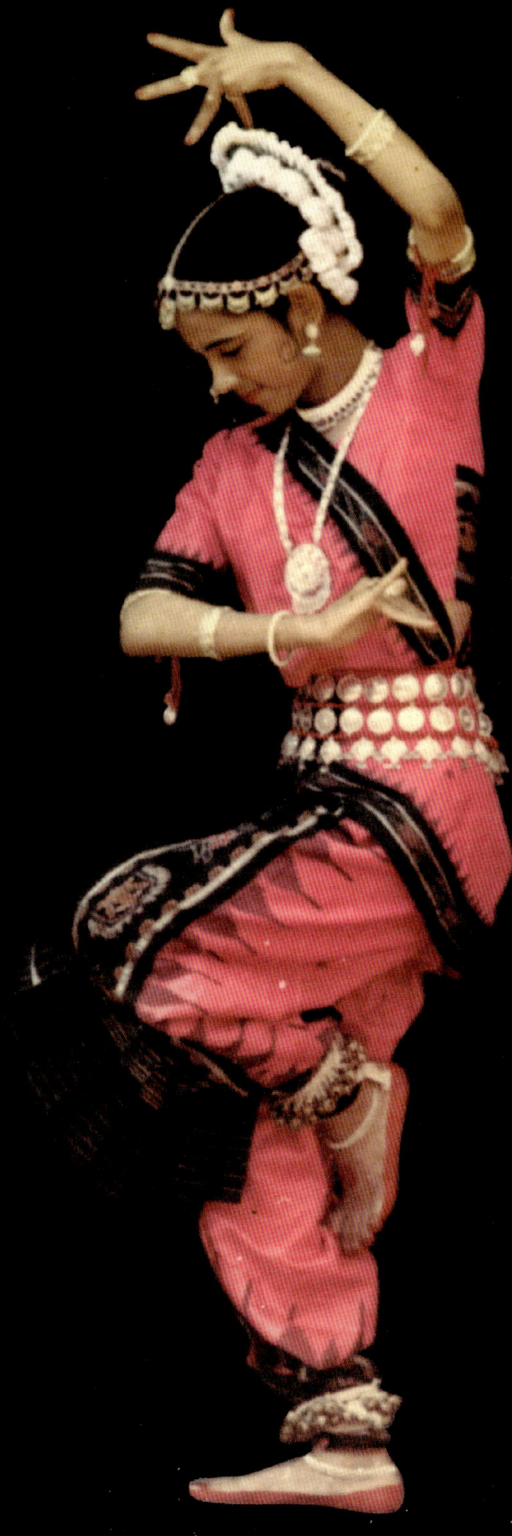

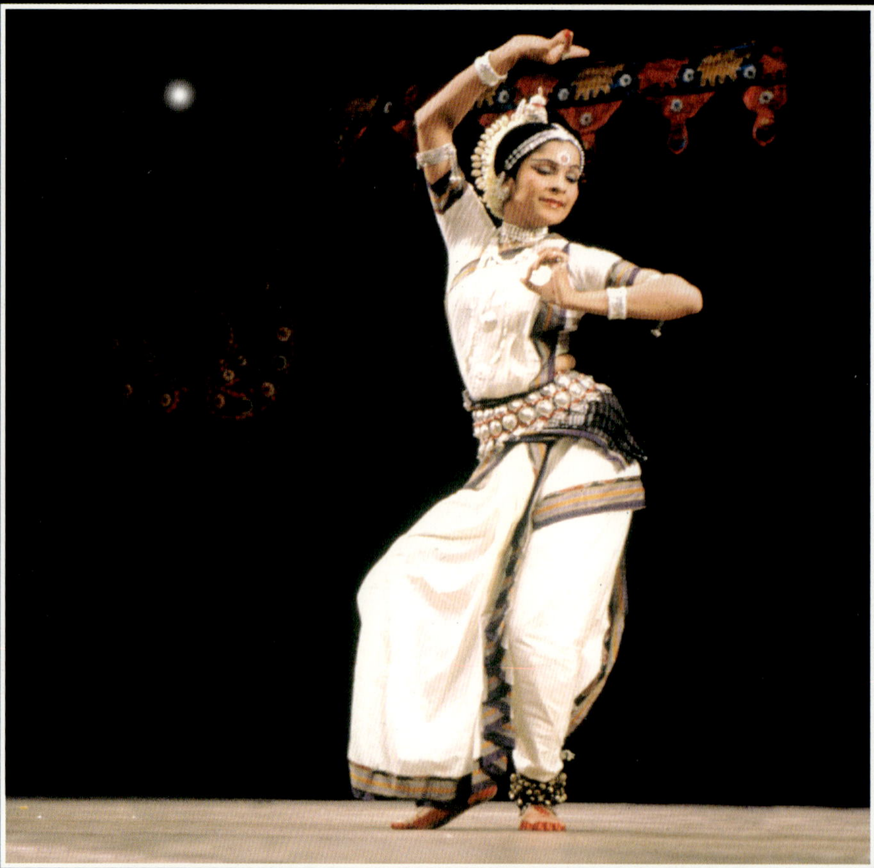

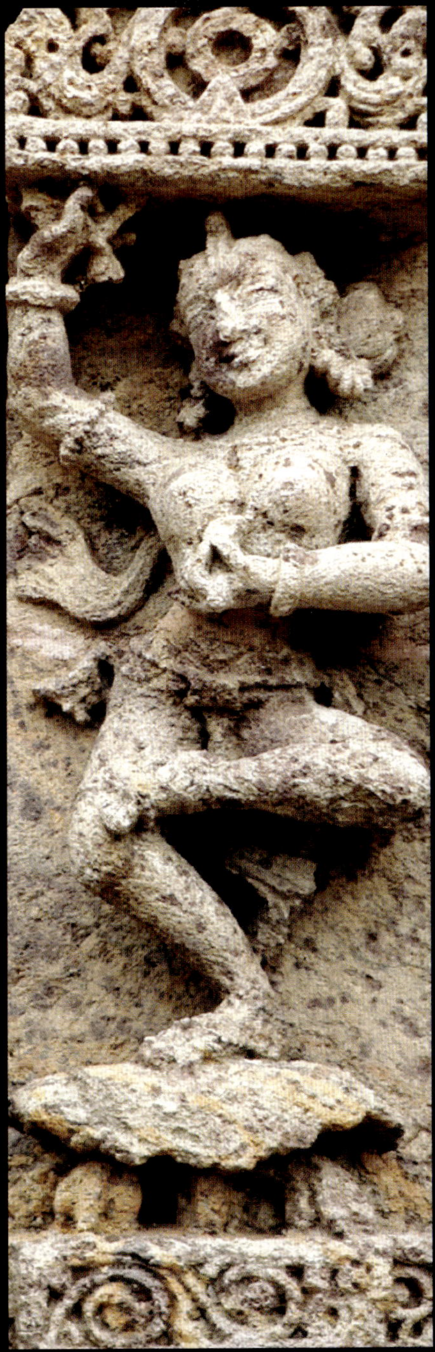

Historical Perspective

Each region occupies a special place in its contribution to the cultural mosaic of the country. This has been specially true for the growth of Indian culture. Indian culture has been expansive and has encouraged the emergence of many regionalistic elements in various artistic fields. Orissa is one of the most picturesque, historically rich and artistically active regions of our country. All through history Orissa has retained a cultural identity much more prominent than its political identity. Political stability and economic viability during certain periods have resulted in spurts of cultural activities. Even within certain periods, particular kings stand out for their active encouragements to art, architecture and other cultural activities. What is important is that while developing itself as a vital part of India, constantly expanding and receding its territorial frontiers according to the power of different rulers, it has also absorbed and has been influenced by the cultural traditions of the neighbouring areas.

The cultural development of any region is conditioned by various geographical factors and Orissa, in that respect, is no exception. The geographical situation of the land has to be considered for shaping its culture. Orissa is like a bridge between the northern and southern halves of the country where the plains of the coastal belt as well as the river belts in various directions have made human contact easier within the country. In addition, its coastal line has provided a gateway for overseas and in the process has exported much of its art and culture to some of the neighbouring countries. Through ages, Orissa has nurtured a rich cultural heritage and has contributed significantly to the cultural development of the country.

The growth of Orissan culture has been expansive from the very beginning. The name Orissa has got superimposed on the grandiose and dignified name of Kalinga which was a mighty political power to reckon with. Ancient and medieval Kalinga saw the rise and fall of some of the most powerful empires and kingdoms from the pre-Christian centuries till the time of its decline in the 16th century. The notable dynasties which ruled over the territory were the Chedi or the Aire Mahameghavahana, the Mathra, the Bhauma-Kara, the Somavansi, the Ganga and the Surya. Art and culture flourished under the powerful dynasties, enjoying patronage of several great kings.

A study of the art, architecture and literature of the region reveals that the art of dance has occupied a special place in the evolution of Orissan culture. Of course, in a greater perspective, dance evolved in intimate association with the development of dance tradition in the country. The *Natyashastra* of Bharata Muni, which is the earliest surviving text on dance and drama, classifies these arts into four regional types, namely *Avanti, Dakshinatya, Panchali* and *Odra-Magadhi.* According to some texts, *Odra-Magadhi* style was practiced in Anga, Vanga, Kalinga, Vatsa, Odhra, Magadha, Pundra and some other eastern regions of India. Out of these, it would be safe to say that Kalinga and Odhra evidently refer to the present-day Orissa. Thus, a *shastric* tradition in dance existed in Orissa around the second century BC, the time of *Natyashastra.*

Dance has always been an important motif for the ornamental sculpture in Indian temples and is also indicative of the dance tradition of the time. Orissa is exceptionally rich, both in temples and in dance sculptures so much so that many people opine that the tradition of Odissi dance has been preserved in the temple architecture. Prevalence of dance figures in the temples also reflect the close relationship between dance and religion.

The earliest surviving edifices in Orissa are the rock-cut cave temples at Khandagiri and Udayagiri. These shrines were made for Jaina recluses. The first inscriptional evidence for the tradition of dance and music is found in the *Hati Gumpha* of Udayagiri built by the Jain king Maharaja Kharavela in 2nd century BC. According to the inscriptions, King Kharavela himself has been referred to as *Gandharva-veda-budha* meaning an expert in *Gandharva,* which is a synonym for music. The inscriptions further indicate that during the third year of his rule, King Kharavela organised a show by the music-dance-drama experts for the entertainment of the general public. This is the first inscriptional reference to the art of music-dance-drama in Orissa and even in India. This inscription has been translated into Sanskrit by Rajguru (1978):

Trutiye Punarvarse Gandharva-Veda-Budhah Darpa
Nrutta-Gita-Vaditra Sandarshaneirutshabah
Samajakaranavishchha Kritayati nagarim.

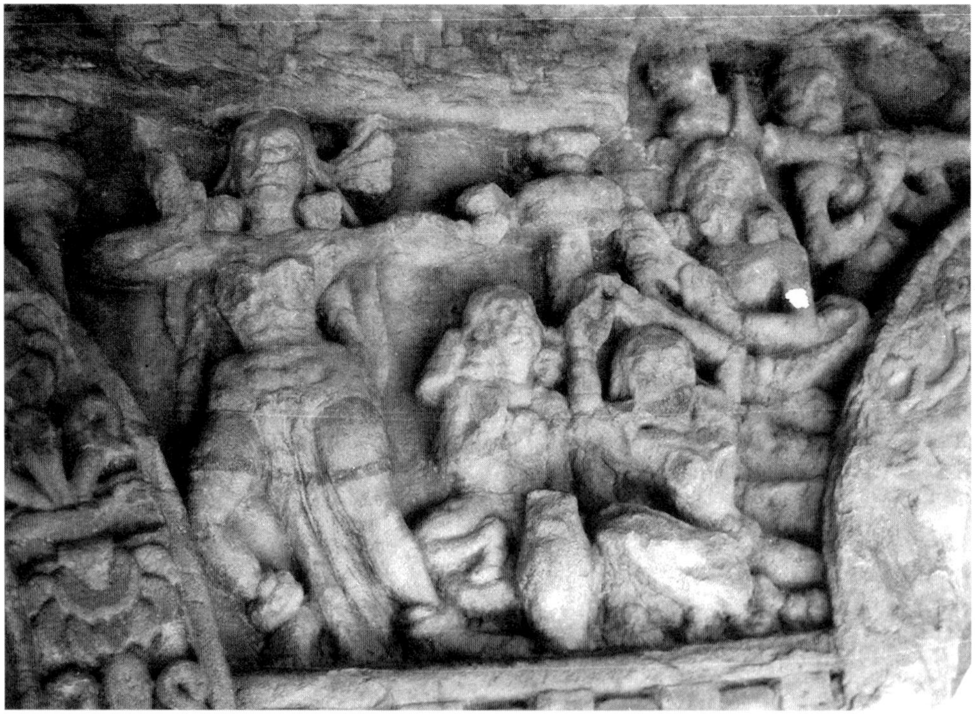

Dancer with musicians, Hatigumpha cave.

Besides the rock edicts, there are a number of panels depicting music and dance. On the right side of the *Rani Gumpha* cave in Udayagiri, a group of men and women devotees are seen engaged in singing and dancing around a *chaitya* tree to the accompaniment of musical instruments such as the *veena, mardala,* flute and cymbals. In the *Rani Gumpha* is present a frieze of considerable significance. Between two false arches is a representation of a danseuse performing in front of the *neptyagriha*, accompanied by an orchestra consisting of two women drummers, one male harpist and one male flutist. The movement is well caught and according to Fabri (1974), can be looked upon as the earliest representation of Odissi dance. In addition, one sees *Gandharvas*, *Vidyadharas* and female figures carved in beautiful postures.

A study of art and architecture during the post-Kharavela period gives evidence to the fact that dance provided the inner rhythms of harmony of Orissan temples. The use of figures in dancing poses in the architecture is also indicative of the fact that dance art has caught the imagination of people of Orissa through ages. As in other parts of India, dance has been intimately associated with religion in Orissa. This is not surprising as dancing is perhaps the most ancient of arts and, in itself, is considered to be a religion where worship is done through mime, gesture and the rhythm of dancing feet. Specific *mudras* during the *puja* is used from time immemorial by the priests. Therefore, it is not surprising that dance became a part of the ritual as a mode of worship and dancers and musicians, collectively called *devadasis*, were dedicated to deities.

The history of ritualistic association of dance and music in Orissa has to be considered in the light of the religious traditions prevalent during the different periods. In the post-Kharavela era, from the 3rd century AD, Buddhism began to flourish and continued for five centuries after which Brahminism gained ascendency. Mahayana Buddhism was patronized and encouraged by the Bhauma and Kara kings who ruled over Orissa till the later half of the 8th century AD. However, towards the end of this period, the rigid school of Buddhism showed signs of mellowing and transformed into a more worldly and tangible form of Buddhism known as Vajrayana. Vajrayana Buddhism encouraged creative activities all over Orissa, specially the Assia range of hills – Lalitagiri, Udayagiri and Ratnagiri in Jajpur (formerly Cuttack district). The Buddhist-constructed shrines are representative of the dyamic art of this period. The door jambs, grills, lintels and architraves of the shrines often carry carvings which include dance figures of both men and women. By the 6th century, one can see excellent sculptures in clear *tribhanga* (thrice-bent) pose, with beautifully proportioned body carved with elegance and feminine charm in Kosaleswara temple in Bolangir district.

Vajrayana Buddhism contributed to the evolution of a new and enlarged pantheon of Buddhists, embracing several Buddhas, their counter-parts and emanations. What is relevant here is that some of these gods and goddesses have been represented in dance poses. *Heruka, Marichi, Vajravarahi, Achala* and *Aparajita* are some of the Buddhist deities who are represented in dance sculptures in Udayagiri, Lalitagiri, Ratnagiri, Alamgiri, Udla, Khiching, Choudwar, Baudh, Solampur, Ayodhya, Khadipada and Astaranga. Fabri (1974) makes a special mention of an image of a dancer in the sacred precincts of the great monastery at Ratnagiri dated around 850 AD.

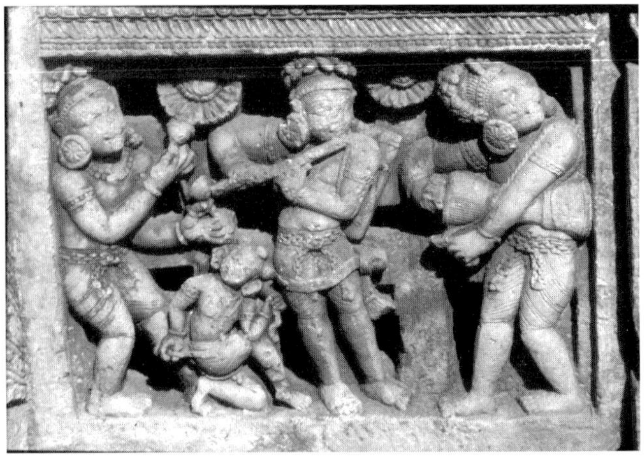

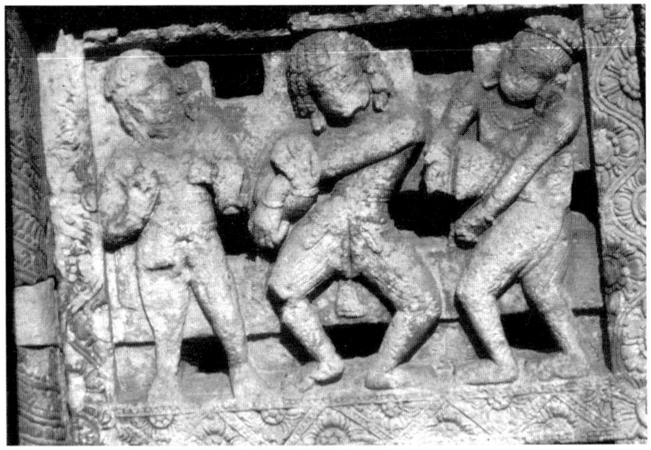

LEFT :
Panel of musicians, Parasurameswar Temple.

RIGHT :
Panel of dancers and musicians, Parasurameswar Temple.

The earliest Hindu temples in Orissa belong to Bhubaneswar and were built around the 7th century AD. After this, temple building began in right earnest in Orissa. However, most of the temples which were built between 7th and 8th centuries are now in ruins, but some of their sculptures and carved panels have been preserved. Among these panels and sculptures are figures of dancers and a noteworthy grill which carries a vigorous figure of *Nataraja*.

The temple of Parasurameswara (7th century AD) is not only the earliest of the well-preserved shrines of Orissa but is also important in the context of evolution of dance tradition in Orissa as it has some of the characteristic Odissi dance poses. The characteristic *chauka* (pose which has four right angles at shoulder, elbow, thigh and knee) position is very well depicted in the form of two dancers. In addition, on the grills, in the front facades of the *Jagamohana,* there are panels of musicians and dancers. The main body of the temple contain some beautiful *tandava* figures.

After this came the period of Bhaumas (8th-9th century AD) and to this period belong two important Shaivite temples – the Vaital Deul and the Sisireswara. Both temples carry a number of interesting dance sculptures. The typical Orissan *alasakanyas* profusely used in the modern day Odissi dance and therefore dealt with detail later, are placed at random along the walls of the temples.

FACING PAGE :
Kandarpa Ratha from Jagannath Temple, Puri.

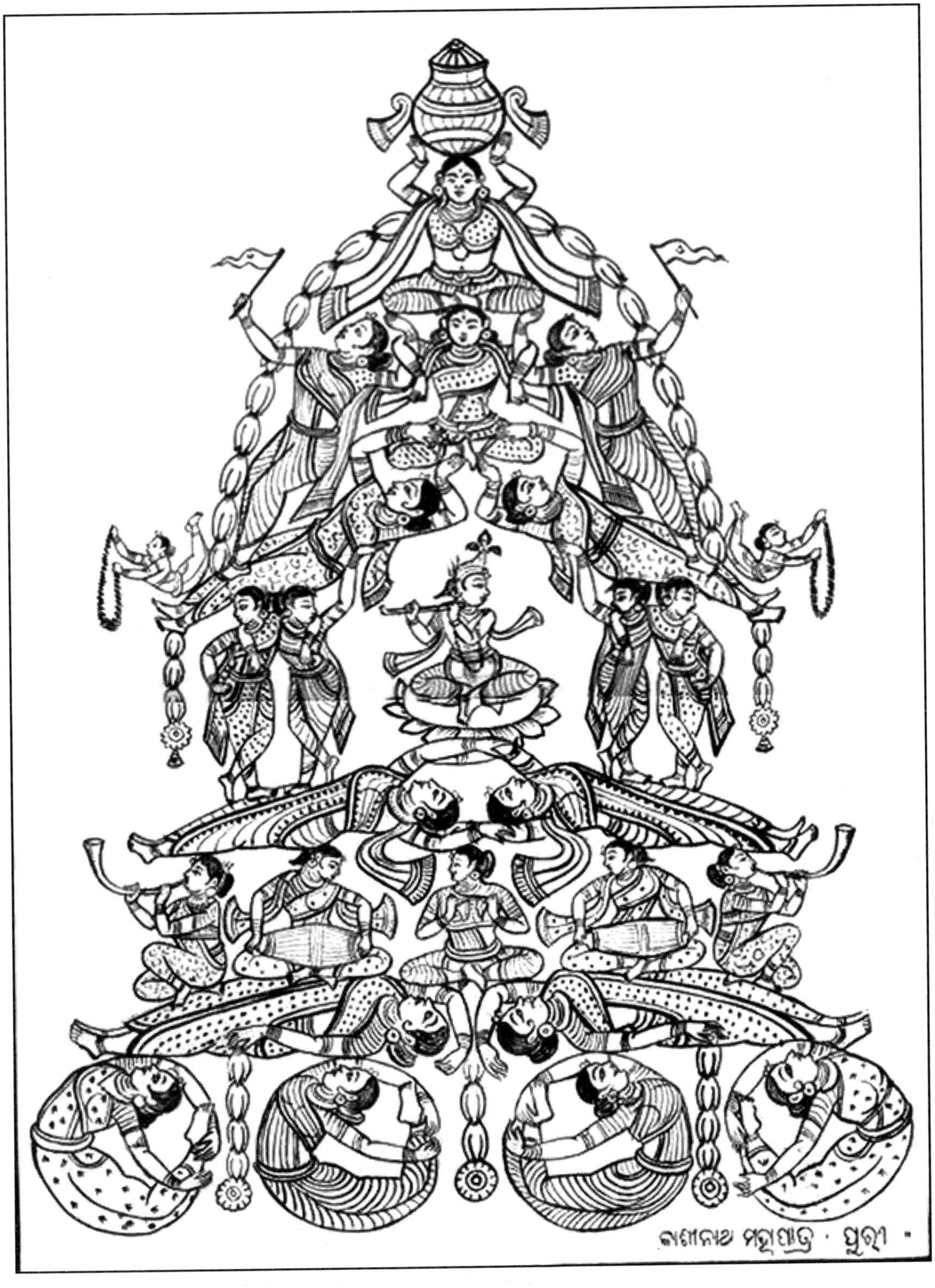
ଜଗନ୍ନାଥ ମହାପାତ୍ର · ପୁରୀ ·

The Vaital Deul has a framed figure of *Nataraja* on the uppermost part of its facade. The Sisireswara also has a *Nataraja*, and close to this is a figure of a *dwarapala* in a graceful pose.

After the Bhauma Period, the Soma or the Kesari dynasty of Mahakosala came into power. The Kesari dynasty ruled up to 11th century till it was replaced by the Ganga rulers. The Kesari rulers were Vaishnavites and later converted to Shaivism. After the Bhauma Period, and up to the time of the construction of Lingaraja temple marking the Kalinga style of architecture, many temples were built in Bhubaneswar which are of much significance. All these temples carry a series of some of the most interesting dance sculptures.

Outstanding amongst these is the Mukteswara (9th century AD) which has been described as a poem in stone. It has several exquisite dance carvings including the figures of *Nataraja, nayikas* and other dancing postures. Many of the dance postures carved in this temple have a striking resemblance to the modern-day Odissi dance poses. It has several stances of *alasakanyas,* beautiful young girls decorating all the Orissan temples in sculpturesque poses. The sculptor has captured exquisite facial expressions, detailed hair styles, jewellery and clothings in his carvings. In a panel is an eight-armed dancing Ganesha, with a snake held above his head, and his mouse in the front. Two seated musicians are shown, one with drums and the other with cymbals, and there are two dancing *gana* attendants. The four corners of the ceiling are filled with figures of dancers.

The Ananta Vasudeva (13th century AD), which is the only Vaishnava temple of Bhubaneswar, is fairly well decorated with carvings which include dance poses. The Kapileswara temple carries a three-panel frame of dancers and musicians. All the three male dancers are seen in a row in various poses.

During the Ganga rule (12th century AD), a greater emphasis appears to have been placed on the performance of music and dance in religious shrines. This is evident from the fact that a separate hall, the *Natamandapa,* was built for music and dance performances.

The Rajarani temple belongs to the early part of the Ganga Period dated around 10th century AD which carries numerous beautiful dance poses interspersed between columns of floral designs. There are dance sculptures

FACING PAGE :
Konarak: Panel with Dancers.

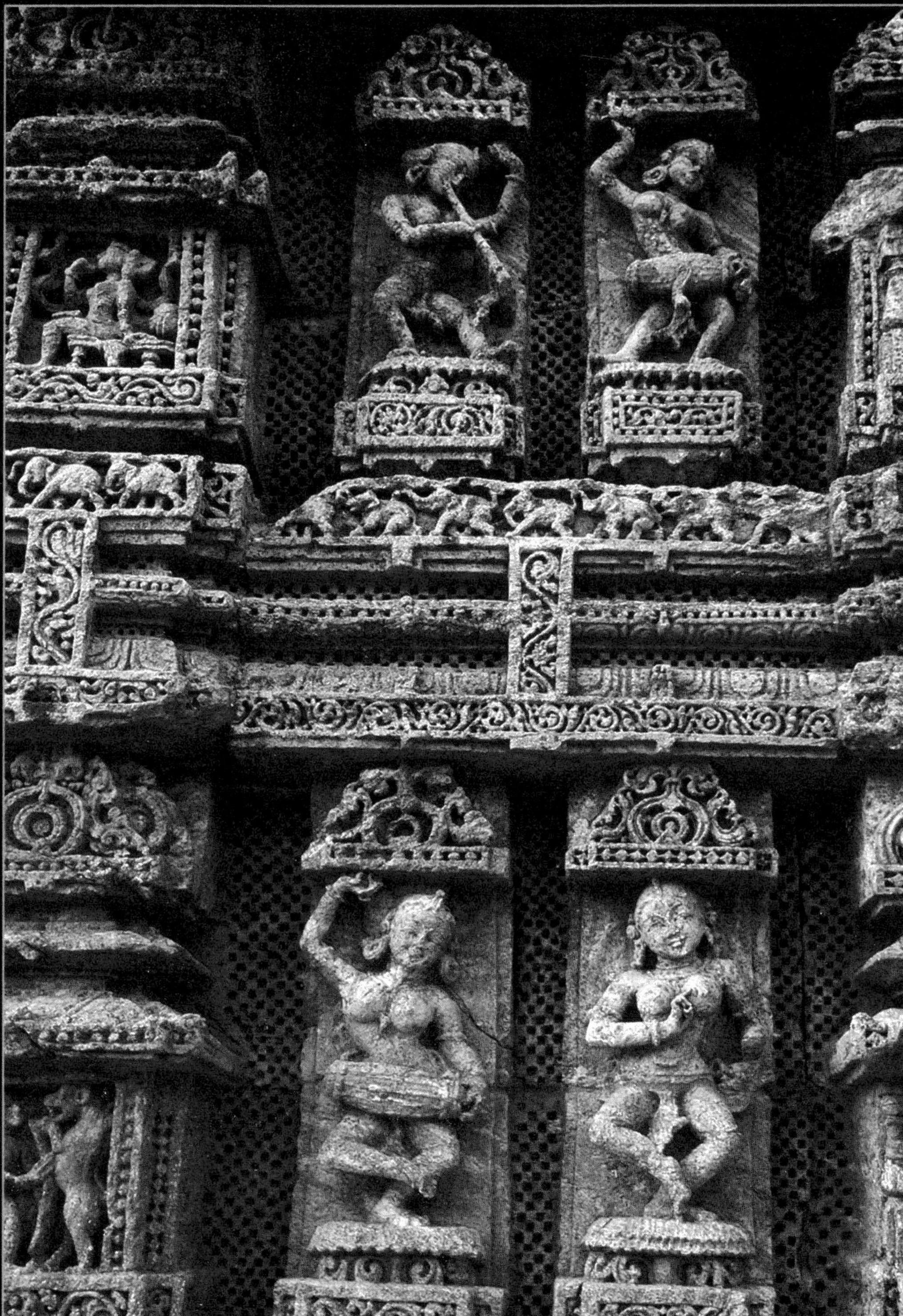

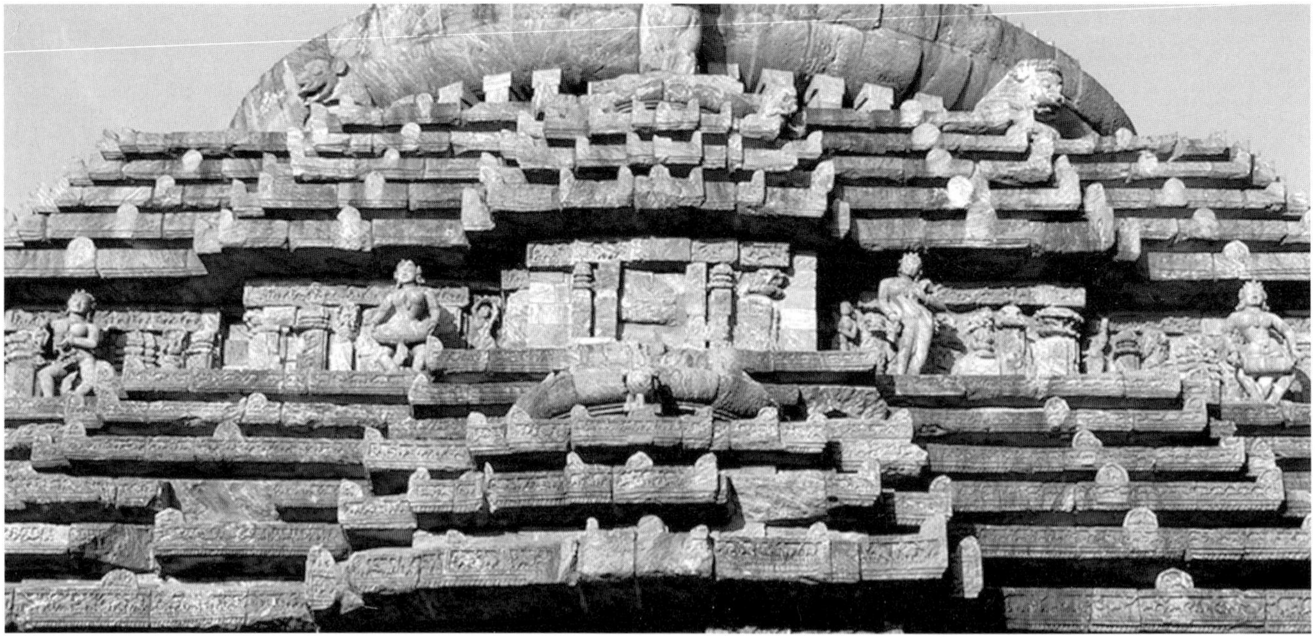

Larger than life statues of Konarak (courtesy: Sadasiba Pradhan)

of *Nataraja, ganas* and other deities as well as those of *Gandharvas.* A panel on the plinth of the temple shows goddess Parvati in a vigorous dance pose. Of her five female attendants, two are seen carrying musical instruments in a dancing posture while rest of the three play on musical instruments. The whole *Vimana* of the temple is lavishly decorated with what Fabri describes as "a forest of ornamentation". In addition to the creepers and scrollwork, there are enchanting *alasakanyas.* Lower down, in miniature frames, as part of the decoration, is a dancing Shiva. To the same period belong two other important temples of Orissa – the Lingaraja in Bhubaneswar and the Jagannath in Puri. Both these temples and their subsidiary shrines are adorned with dance sculptures including *apsaras* and *nayikas*, many of them in typical *alasakanya* pose. Inside the Puri temple is a *Kandarpa Ratha* made up of many female figures in acrobatic poses used in the *bandha nritya* in Odissi. It appears that it is a later addition to the temple but what is important here is that it is a significant sculpture directly relevant to modern-day Odissi dance.

FACING PAGE : *Nrutyaguru with inscription (Saumya Sridatta), Konarak Temple (courtesy: Sadasiba Pradhan).*

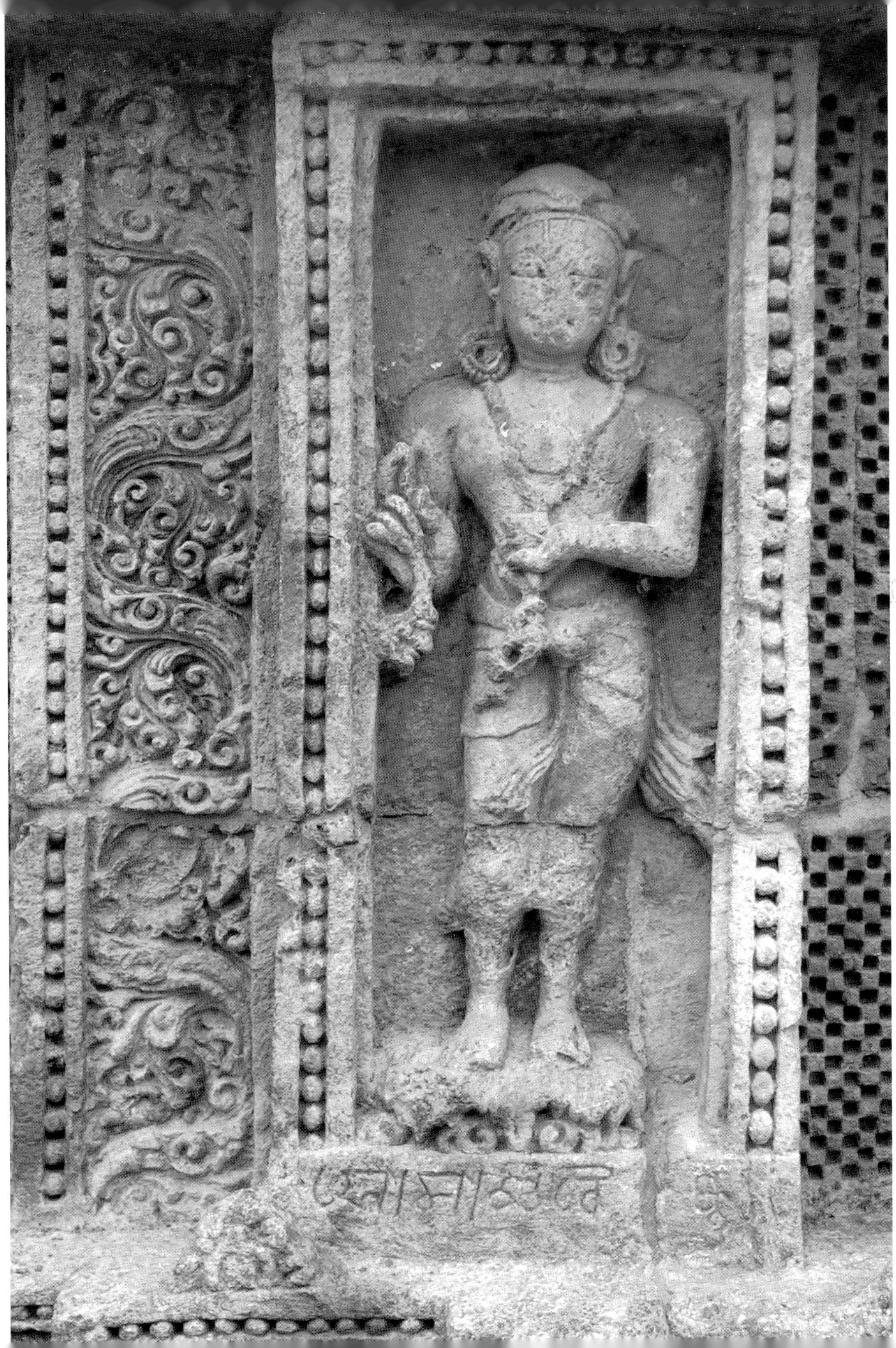

The most important temple to be built around this period was Konarak dedicated to Surya Deva. It was built by the Ganga King Narasimha I around 1250 AD. In the temple of Konarak the whole edifice becomes sculptured and carved. The plinth, the walls and the *Vimana* of *Jagamohana* carry hundreds of carvings of dancers and musicians. Konarak is the only temple in India with larger-than-life-size free standing celestial musicians on the parapet of the roof of the *Jagamohana*, playing musical instruments namely, the *mardala* (drum), *gini* (cymbals) *veena*, *venu* (flute) and *kahali* (a trumphet). Being carved from single piece of stone they are unique of their kind and remind one of the poses used in the *batu nritya* in modern-day Odissi repertoire. The *Natamandapa* of Konarak is situated at a distance of 300 feet from the *Jagamohana*, which is unusual for Orissan temple in which the *Natamandapa* is usually attached to the *Jagamohana*. The entire plinths and pillars of the *Natamandapa* are covered with carvings of dancing girls and musicians. Many of the poses are profusely used in the Odissi dance today. What is of great significance here is the importance that has been given to the *Nrityaguru* of the time. The temple has only one inscription under a male figure (about 2 feet in height in the *Natamandapa*), holding the cymbals in an attitude of almost going to strike the two together. The left hand is in front of the belly and the right hand in a *kapithya mudra*, holding a cymbal. According to Behera (1971, 1996), the inscription was first noticed by Ramachandran in 1950 who read it as "Saumya Sridatta" representing the *Natyacharya* of the period. Subsequently, Behera, an authority on Konarak, has deciphered it as "Somai Vaisna (va)" who could be the dance master as interpreted by Ramachandran. It is generally agreed that it is not only the representation of a famous *Nrityaguru* of the contemporary period but also indicative of the importance given to the art of dance during that time. Needless to say, the artists who conceived and carved the figures in Konarak gave tremendous importance to dance. Details of different types of dance, costumes, jewellery and musical instruments have been discussed by Behera (1996).

FACING PAGE :
Alasakanya, Alasa, Brahmeswar Temple.

A study of the temple sculpture through ages indicates that dance not only supplied the inner rhythms of harmony but also documented the evolution of Odissi dance in stone. Many of the *karanas* listed in the *Natyashastra* and other texts are depicted in the temples of Orissa. If one considers the dance sculptures from the context of modern-day Odissi dance, apart from the dancing figures of deities, one can divide other dance sculptures into broadly two categories: the musicians and the *alasakanyas.* The musicians are found playing various instruments in various dancing stances (Panigrahi, 1961).

There has been the tradition of the use of *alasakanyas* which can be easily seen in the modern-day Odissi dance (Mohanty Hejmadi, 1998). Apparently, they were used as decorative charms to attract the soul of the created towards the creator. In *Silpa Prakasa,* the author recommends its profuse use in the *Vimana* and *Mukhasala* (see Bonner and Rath Sharma, 1966). He states that a temple without this type of decoration will remain without interest and bear no fruit. Altogether, sixteen types are described in the text which have been listed below.

***Alasa* (the indolent):** A very common posture where on the left side of the middle line is the head. The arms are placed above the head, the hip being deflected to the left side. The right leg is bent and the left leg held at an oblique. Often a variation in the leg position is found with the legs crossed. There are two variations of this pose–*chandita* (palms turned upwards) and *spandita* (palms turned downwards).

***Torana* (leaning on the doorway):** The figurine is turned to the right side. The arm lies in the oblique. The *torana* holds one hand in

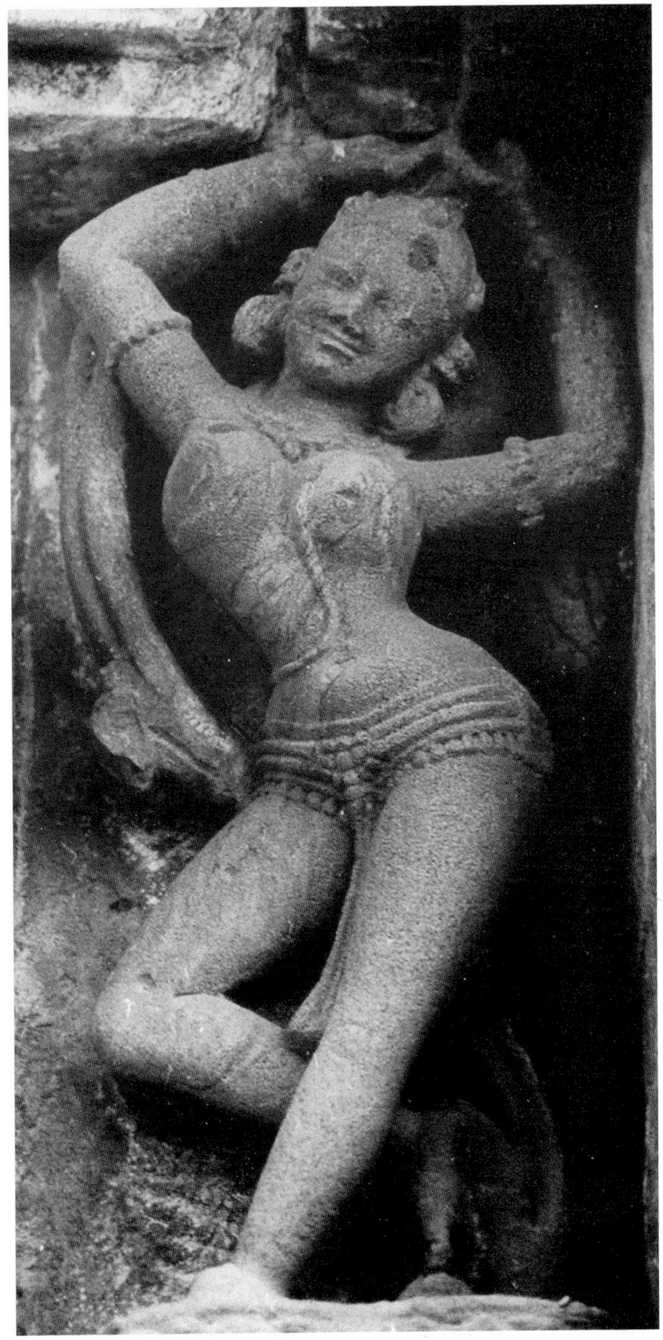

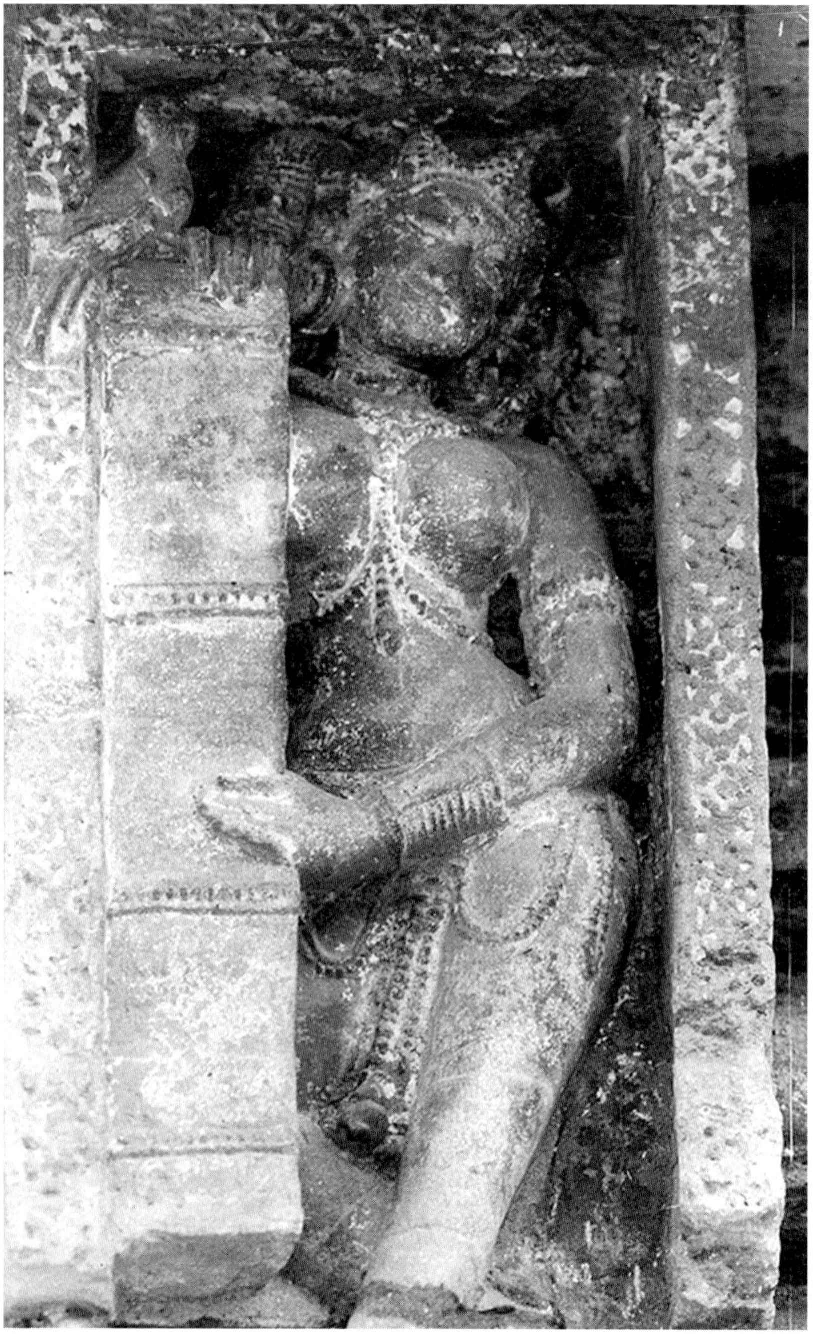

spandita mudra. This figure is found partly hidden by the door against which it is leaning. A considerable variety is found in terms of figures – heavy at Parasurameswara to more shapely ones at Mukteswar, from a few inches to 2-3 feet in height.

***Mugdha* (innocent, simple girl):** The innocent maiden adorned with all the ornaments has one hand in the *nagasira mudra* in front of the face. The *nagasira mudra* is on the right, the left arm is along the line, hip is deflected to one side, the two legs are slanting towards the right side like those of *spandita-alasa*.

***Manini* (resentful or offended girl):** The head is turned towards the left side, the right arm is above the head, with one palm on the head, the left is on the lower lip. The left leg is straight and the right leg is bent, the shank is bent backwards touching the wall. The emphasis is more on the mood where both eyes are half opened and on the lips there is a mood of love *(lasya-bhaba)*.

***Dalamalika* (garlanding herself with a branch):** The head is in a profile, the right forearm goes along with the branch. Hip is deflected to the side. The left upper

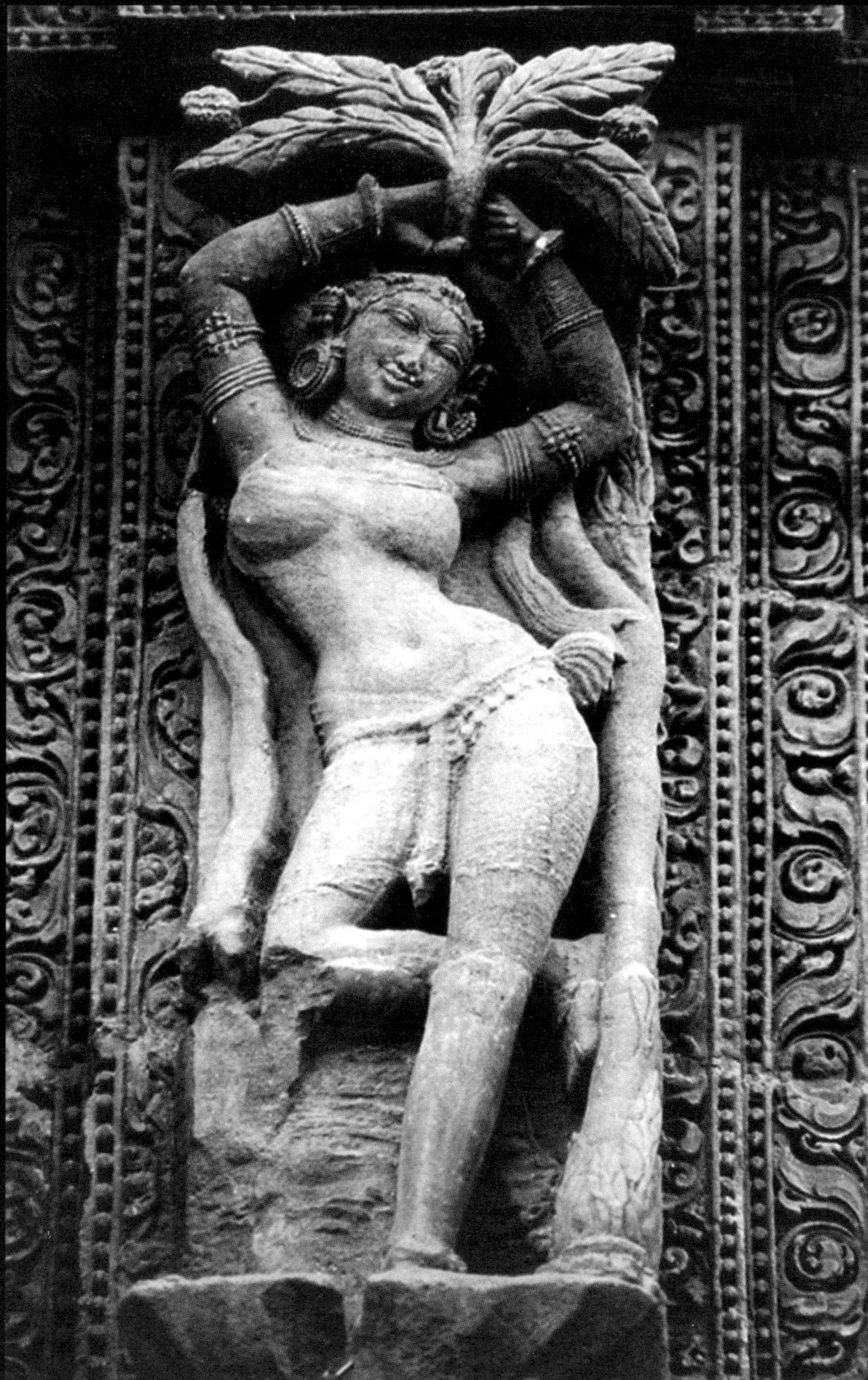

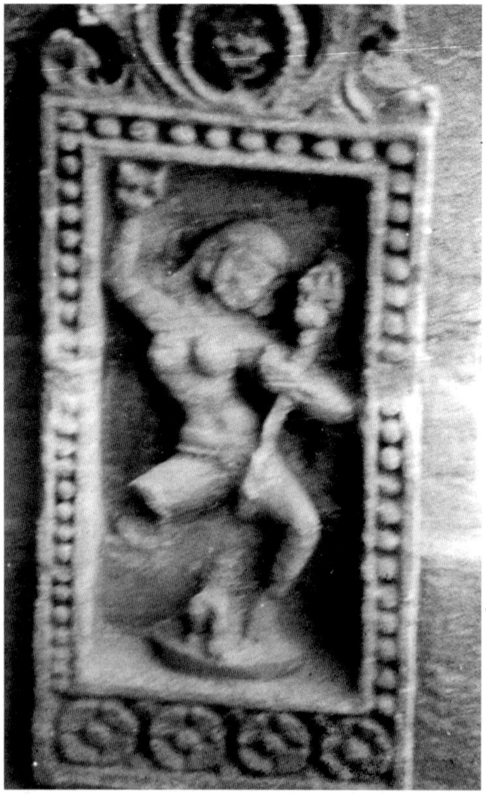

Alasakanya, Padmagandha, Rajarani Temple.

arm is bent downwards and the forearm is bent upwards, touching the end of the branch. The right leg goes across with the left leg which is held straight.

***Padmagandha* (smelling the lotus):** She enjoys the fragrance of the lotus and therefore is known as *padmagandha*. Turned to the left, the head, trunk and the legs are elegantly poised. The left upper arm is on the side. Lying along the forearm bent upwards, she holds a fresh beautiful lotus in her left arm. The right arm is held straight down, resting on the hip. The right leg is slightly slanting and the lower part touches the wall. The left leg is held straight.

***Darpana* (holding a mirror):** The left arm is raised above the head and the palm is placed on the hair towards the front. Her looks are turned down towards the right side of *madhya-rekha* (mid-line). The right forearm goes downwards and the upper arm is bent upwards, holding the mirror *(darpana)*. The right leg goes down to the left corner, the left thigh crosses over with the leg placed on the oblique. Considerable variations are seen with the mirror being held in front of her face in various ways. In some, the right leg crosses over to the left also.

***Vinyasa* (having her mind fixed on meditation):** The girl is turned to the right and her lovely face is seen in profile. The two arms are close to the shoulders (body). The left arm is along the left side, the forearm crossing in front along the horizontal mid-line. The other arm is in the same position and the palm is placed in *karakacchapika* (small tortoise) *mudra*. The left leg is held straight. The right leg is held at an angle with the hands poised in *japanyasa*, *vinyasa* lost in meditation.

***Ketakibharana* (wearing *ketaki* blossom):** On the left side are the head, chest, hip and arm. The right arm is raised, the forearm goes to mid-line. The palm is placed on the left side of her head. The hand holds a *ketaki* leaf. The hip is deflected to the left. The left hand is folded up, with the hand holding a flower. The left leg is held at the oblique with the right leg crossing it at the back *(chandita pada)*.

PRECEDING PAGES :

PAGE 14 :
Alasakanya, Torana, Mukteswar Temple.

PAGE 15 :
Alasakanya, Dalamalika, Rajarani Temple.

FACING PAGE :
Alasakanya, Darpana, Konarak Temple.

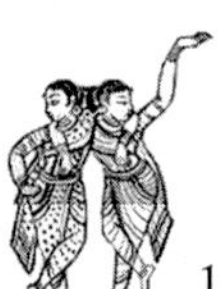

***Matrumurti* (image of mother):** The whole body, including the head, is placed upon the midline. The child is on the left side, held by the mother. Both the legs are held in an ordinary natural position, the hip deflected slightly to hold the weight of the child.

***Camara* (holding a fly whisk):** She is an attendant of the deities. The head is turned towards the right or left. On her right (or left) arm, she holds the *camara* (fly whisk). With the other hand, she holds her garment. According to *Silpa Prakasa*, the legs and feet are in positions similar to those of *Matrumurti*, but in the sculptures the legs are also crossed with the left leg on the oblique and the right crossing over to the left in *chandita pada.*

***Gunthana* (hiding herself):** *Gunthana* is a woman concealing herself with a veil, always showing her back in three bends *(tribhanga)*. The head is straight in the middle. The left arm is in front of the body, touching the lower lip. The right arm is raised up and folded over the head. She stands in a virile attitude *(virasana).* At times she holds a drapery of flowers, and at others, a fan.

***Nartaki* (dancer):** This is the most common sculpture in Konarak. The *Nartaki* turns her body and looks towards the right side. The head is above and the arms are raised towards the sky. Above, the hands are joined with interlocked fingers *(chanda palli)* on the middle vertical. The hip is placed on the right side. The right leg goes down to the left lower corner. The left leg crosses *(chanda)* behind and is placed on the ground.

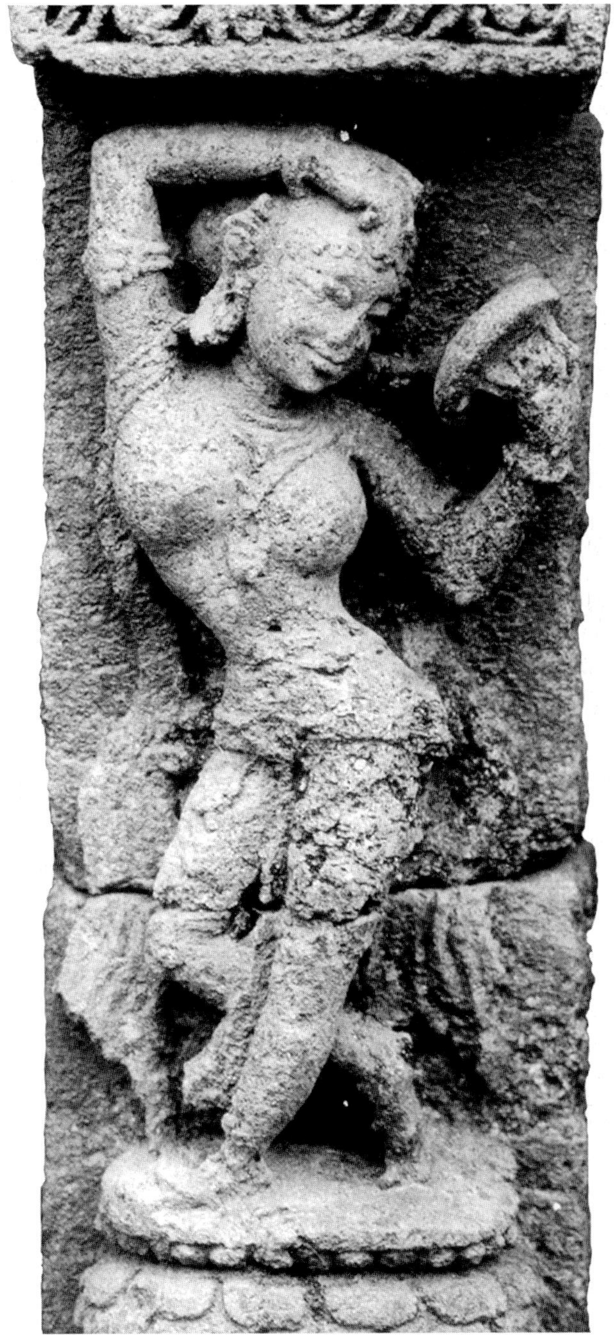

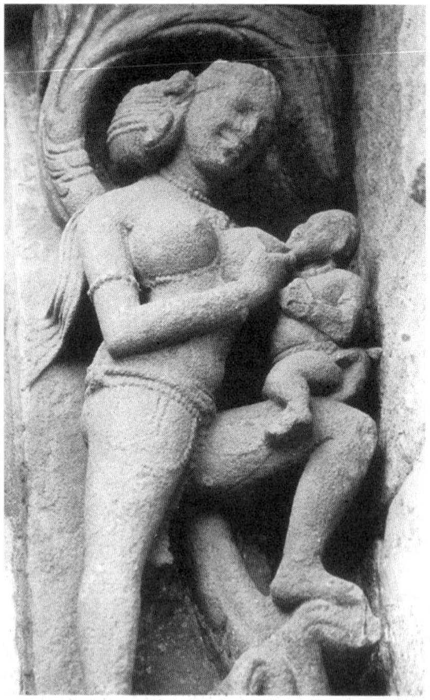 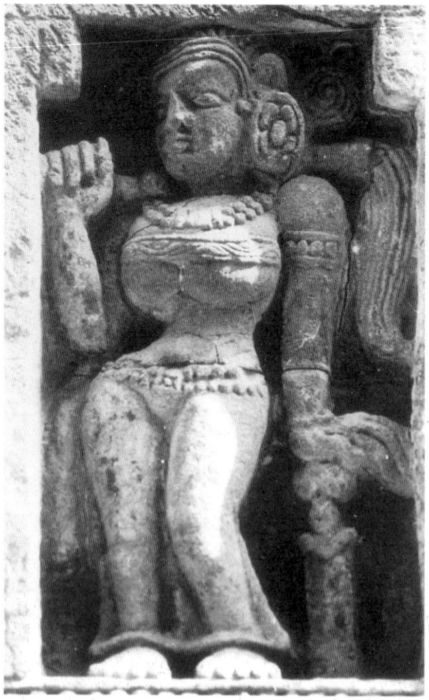 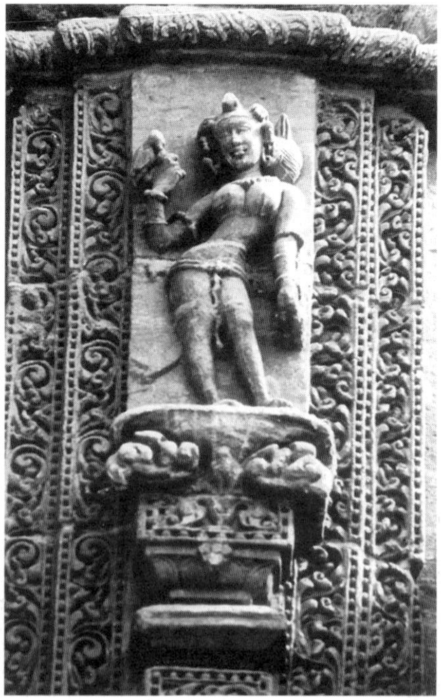

LEFT :
Alasakanya, Matrumurti, Brahmeswar Temple.

CENTRE :
Alasakanya, Camara, Parasurameswar Temple.

RIGHT :
Alasakanya, Sukasarika, Rajarani Temple.

FACING PAGE :
Alasakanya, Mardala, Konarak Temple.

***Sukasarika* (playing with a parrot or a *maina*):** The head is bent to the left side. The right arm is raised up with which she holds a parrot or a *maina* or other beautiful birds. Both legs are in a slanting position, the left shank turned towards the wall, the whole body resting on the right leg.

***Nupurapadika* (with ankle bells):** The body is turned to the right or left. The left or right arm hangs down. The right arm resembles that of *sukasarika* and holds a flower bud. The right or left leg is bent, the knee touching the first horizontal. The shank is placed obliquely towards the left or right side. The left or right hand is placed where there is a string of ankle-bells, her finger-tips are on the ankle bells. The other leg is slanting down to the end of the mid-line.

***Mardala* (drummer):** The head is slightly bent to the left. A *mardala* is placed below the waist. The arms go down with the two arms placed on the *mardala*. The left foot rests on the ground, the right foot is at the same place along the mid-line. This is the beautiful *mardala*, intoxicated with her play.

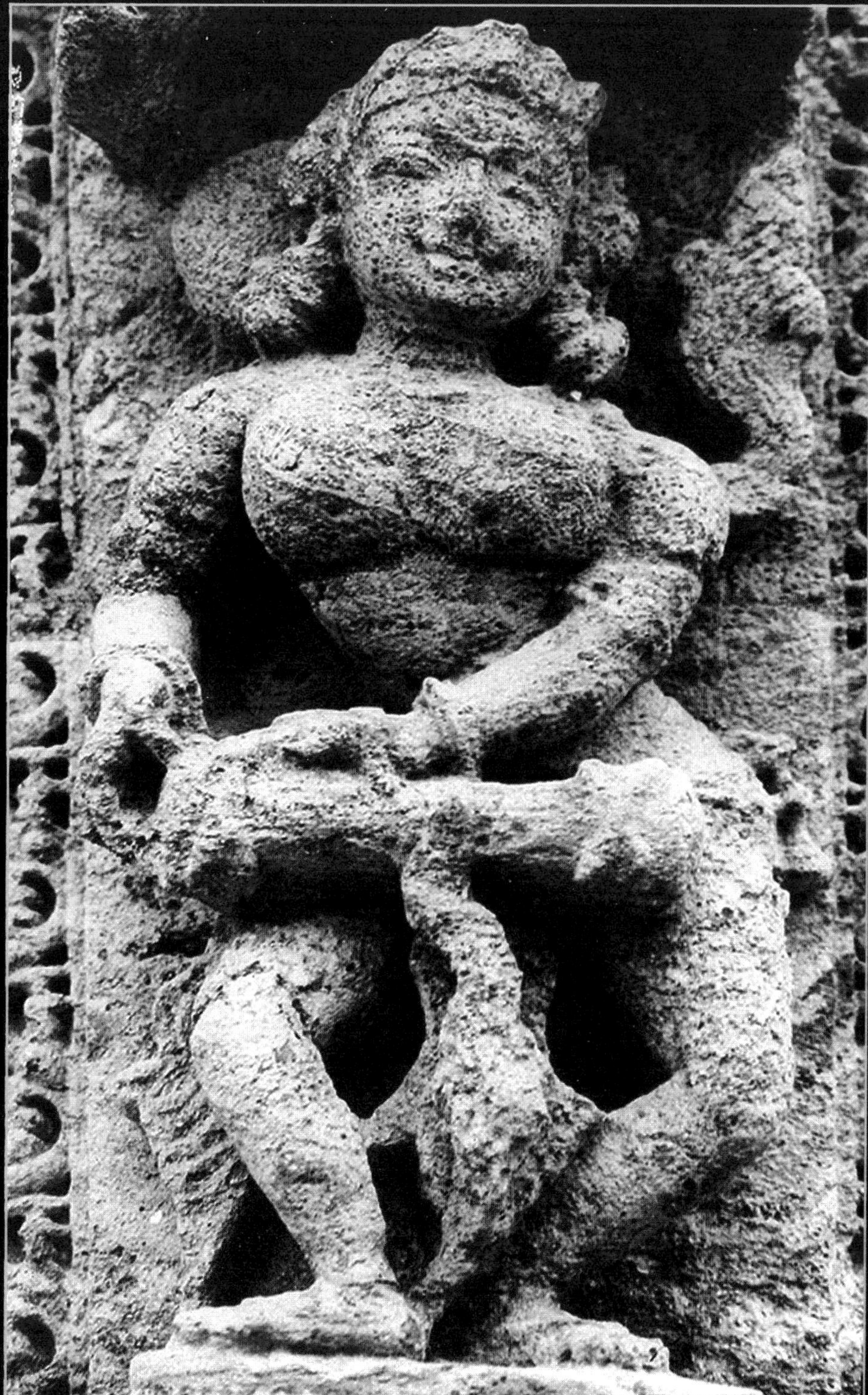

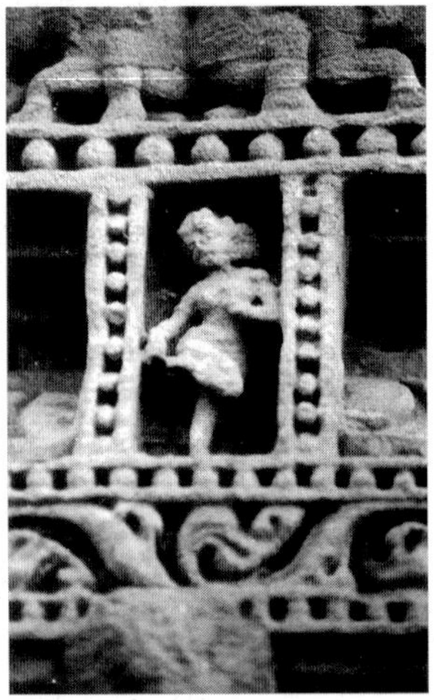

Alasakanya, Nupurapadika, Rajarani Temple.

What is interesting is that one sees *alasakanyas* from the Brahmeswar temple culminating in their profuse use in Konarak. In Konarak, one can already see the permutations and combinations of different types of *alasakanyas* and some deviations from the text of *Silpa Prakasa* regarding the positions of head, torso and legs representative of some artistic freedom that is bound to come with time and creativity.

REFERENCES

Behera, K.S., 1971. "Two Inscriptions from Konarak", *Bharati*-Utkal University Journal - *Humanities*, Vol V (9): 39-47.

—–, 1996. *Konarak – The Heritage of Mankind*, 2 vols., Aryan Books International, New Delhi.

Bonner, Alice and Sadasiva Rath Sharma, 1966. *Silpa Prakasa of Ramachandra Kaulacara* (translated and annotated), Leiden.

Fabri, C., 1974. *History of the Art of Orissa*, Orient Longman Ltd., New Delhi.

Mohanty Hejmadi, Priyambada, 1998. *Odissi Dance*, Nagsbund Foundation for Art and Culture, New Delhi.

Panigrahi, K.C., 1961. *Sculptural Representations of Music and Dance in Orissa,* Souvenir, Fifth All India Youth Hostels Conference.

Rajguru, Satyanarayana, 1978. *Odisare' Sangitara Aitihasikavitti*, Seminar on Odissi Dance (in Oriya), Orissa Sangeet Natak Academy, pp. 50-55.

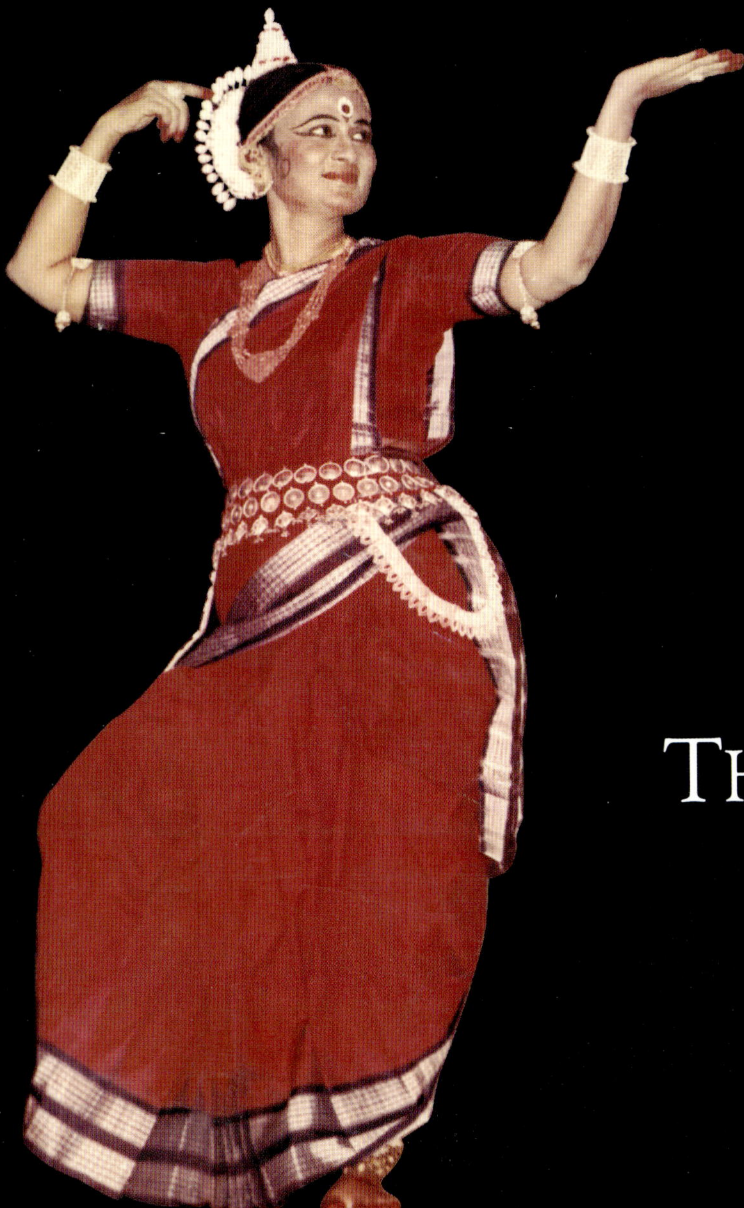

THE PARAMPARA 2

It has been rightly said that the present-day Odissi dance owes its origin to the ritualistic dance practice of the *maharis* in temples and the establishment of *gotipua* system for entertainment outside the temples. The two systems have been briefly discussed by Pattanaik (1974). In this chapter, further details are presented on these two important traditions.

THE MAHARIS

As in other parts of India, in Orissa also dance came to be closely connected with religion. Dance was considered as a mode of worship and dancers as well as musicians *(devadasis)* were dedicated to the deities. It is not known when this practice found its origin in Orissa. According to an article (Anonymous, 1912), it has been found that the system is probably the oldest in India and the author says that, the *devadasis* belonged to Orissa and that they were the chronological successors of the Budhistic *Sthaviras* or *Theras.* The present-day *devadasis* of Puri temple are referred to as *maharis.* Interestingly enough, one hardly finds any documentary evidence of the name *mahari* and even the "Record of Rights" (1952) (Appendix 1), for Puri temple refers to them as *Bhitara gauni (devadasi).* However, one finds the name *mahari* in *Chhamu-Chitau* from Puri Raja's *Diwan* (Mahapatra, 1988 and also one issued in 1886 AD, see Appendix 2). Later, in an article dated 1912 entitled "Deva Dasis" (Anonymous, 1912), they have been referred to as *ma-iri's.* Dr. K.S. Behera (personal communication) feels that the 11th-century Ratnagiri plate of the Somavamsi king also mentions *mahari* as discussed later in this chapter.

In this context, the definitions of *Mahattaris* (Matrons) in *Natyashastra* (see Ghose, undated) may be mentioned. According to this definition, women, who for the protection of the entire harem and for (the king's) prosperity, take pleasure in singing hymns (to Gods), and in performing auspicious ceremonies, are known as *Mahattaris* (Matrons). But its relation to the present-day nomenclature, *mahari* seems remote.

Evidences dating back to the 11th century show clear evidence that the *devadasis* were employed in the Brahmeswar temple. The Brahmeswar temple was constructed during period of Udyota Kesari in the later half of 11th century AD. According to an inscription (*sloka* 15, Gargabatu, 1933) in the emple, Udyota Kesari's mother, Rani Kolavati, had dedicated several beautiful irls to Lord Brahmeswar. The *sloka* further describes the beauty of these irls. Thus, the *Shaivites* had established *devadasi* system in their rituals (Rajguru, undated).

Even the Buddhist Viharas had *devadasis.* The Ratnagiri charter of the Somavamsi king, Karna Deva (11th century), refers to Rani Karpurasri who hailed from Solanapura Mahavihara. She is described as the daughter of Udayamati.

In the Ratnagiri plates of Somavamsi Karna in the 2nd plate; 2nd side, lines 41-48 say that this grant is issued with libations or water free of taxes, for the increase of merit and glory of (our) mother, father (and) ourselves, to Rani Sri Karpurasri, daughter of Maharima Hunadevi and grand-daughter of Udayamati of *Kashyapa gotra* (and) the *pravara* of three *rishis* who migrated from the Mahavihara of Solanapura in Utkaladesa. Let this grant be continued as long as the moon, the sun (and) the earth would endure.

But Prof. K.S. Behera opines (personal communication) that the word "Maharima" is actually "Mahari" and it should be read as "Rani Sri Karpurasri" daughter of "*Mahari* Mahunadevi" instead of "Maharima Hunadevi" and "grand-daughter of Udayamati", consistent with the mother-to-daughter lineage – a practice among the *maharis* till present day.

During the Ganga Period (1114-1435 AD), *devadasi* system became an integral part of the temple organisation. Towards the end of the 12th century, Swapneswar Deva, a relation of Ganga king, Rajaraja Deva II, built the Megheswara temple. In the Megheswara inscription one finds reference to the *devadasis,* interestingly enough to their dance for the first time:

> *The ones whose eyes can enchant the world,*
> *whose foot movements can make the three worlds*
> *(Heaven, Earth and Under-World) stand still,*
> *whose bracelets studded with jewels shine like*
> *Ajanta lamp during their dance,*
> *These doe-eyed girls were dedicated to the*
> *Conquerer of the three worlds – Lord Shiva.*
>
> (Translation of the inscription Megheswara)

During the time of Anangavima Deva (1190-1198 AD), King Baidyanathan built the Shovaneswara temple. An inscription in the temple described the dance and music tradition during that time.

During Ganga dynasty, the capital of Kalinga was Kalinganagara near the river Bansadhara; and "Mukhalinga" and "Srikurma" were the leading *Shaiva* and *Vaishnava* centres for worship, respectively. *Devadasis* or *devaganikas* were employed at these temples for daily rituals. According to an inscription in the Mukhalinga temple – Maharaja Chodaganga Deva had appointed two daughters of *Nrutyaguru* Purnakoti as *devaganika* and two brothers of Purnakoti as *vadyakara* and *gayaka* in the temple and had donated land to two *devaganikas* and *vadyakaras* who were permanently attached to the temple (Rajguru, 1977, 1978). Thus, there are evidences that in Kalinga, the tradition of dedicating *devaganikas, vadyakaras* (musicians) and *gayakas* existed even before the 12th century. They were from the *Vaishya* class and the *devaganikas* were referred to as *gosthi* or *sampradaya* or *mela*. Further, each *sampradaya* was specialized in a particular branch of music and the outstanding ones from each *sampradaya* were rewarded in the *Raja durbar*.

In the Kurmeswar temple, an inscription in Telugu dated around 1252 AD, states that the Ganga king, Vira Narsimha Deva-I, had in 1250 AD dedicated 13 *Sanis* (referred to as *Narasingha Deva Sampradayas*), for performing dance, drama and music in the temple. Out of these, six were for playing the *mardala,* two for dance, one for *pakhawaj*, one for playing the *mahuri* (a type of bugle), one for *Shythin* (difficult to correlate), and one was the *Malangyaka* (can be interpreted as the head of the group). Since in the present time *mardala* and *pakhawaj* are synonyms here, the former may be interpreted as *murdanga (khol)*.

There is evidence that the royal family members practised the art of dance, drama and music. According to the inscriptions in the Ananta Vasudeva temple which was built by the daughter of Anangavima Deva II, Chandrika Devi, in memory of her late husband, Chandrika Devi herself was learned in the *Gita-Laya-Tala* and *Nartana Kala*.

It is generally agreed that the dance ritual in the Jagannath temple which has direct relationship to modern Odissi dance, was started by Anantavarman Chodaganga or Choraganga Deva. Das (1958) makes an interesting speculation regarding the fact that Chodaganga Deva was a connoisseur of dance. According to him, in the year 1067 AD, Anantavarman Choraganga Deva of the Ganga dynasty of Kalinga (then south of Ganjam) came and became the over-lord of the coastal regions, including the place of Purushottam or Jagannath. According to his own inscriptions, he ruled for 72 years. He was a great king with great conceptions, and was a patron of culture and religion. He had a liberal mind and although traditionally a *Shaivite*, his patronage of Vaishnavism is legendary. Besides the Puroshottam (Jagannath) temple at Puri, he constructed Vishnu temples at Mukhalingam, Srikarman and Simachalam.

In describing the clever incorporation of the legends regarding the establishment of *Nilamadhaba* and the image of neem-wood called *Savarinarayana* to the story of the building of the great temple, Das says:

> it seems now certain that Choraganga in the *puranas* became Indradyumna and the sage Ramanuja became Narada. Choraganga, it may be remembered, had a great weakness for women and dancing girls .... Indradyumna has strongly been described to have been surrounded by not only numberless young ladies of the Harem, but also by dancing girls who were in intervals exhibiting their art to please Raja Indradyumna himself. Even the gods are being worshipped by youthful and beautifully over-sexed public girls (Das, 1958).

In any case, it is generally agreed that Choraganga Deva established the *Devadasi* or *Devaganika pratha* (tradition) in Jagannath temple from 12th century which flourished in later times. The details have been described in a Telugu manuscript entitled *Jagannath Sthala Brutantam*. This is apparently a Telugu retranslation of the *Madala Panji*, preserved in the Oriental Manuscript Library of Madras (Rajguru, 1978).

According to the manuscript:

> 24 *Veshyas* (Sani or Maharani), according to Nijoga (assignment), were divided into two groups "Sampradayas" of about 12 each. Each group consisting of both males and females were to assign "nrutya-gita-vadya seva" in Shri Jagannath Mahapravu's 3 daily *dhupas* (meals), *barasinghar* (evening dressing ritual) and *puspanjali* as well as performances at other festivals (*Jatras*) and celebrations (*Utsabs*). In Chandan Jatra, during the Chapa boating of Mahaprabhu, they performed "nrutya-gita and vadya". The music performed during this period

should be of high order according to *shastric* tradition. Furthermore, the ritual is mentioned in the *Skandha Purana* where it is written that:

"ବେଣୁ ବୀଣାଦିବାଦ୍ୟୈଶ୍ଚ ତଥା ନାଦୋପହାରକୈଃ
ସନ୍ତୋଷୟନ ଜଗନ୍ନାଥଂ ତୃତାୟାଦୌଦ ବିଲେପୟତ"

In other words, the dancers and musicians appointed for temple duty were highly proficient in their skills. In addition, 10 *Tanpura* players and fourteen musicians for playing other musical instruments were employed for temple services. The musical performance used to be held near the door of Jagamohana. In addition, there was a special *seva* called *Bhitara-gauni* where specific songs were to be sung according to *shastric* tradition. They were also to be faultless as far as *swara, laya* and *tala* were concerned. An instrument called "reba" – a type of *mukhavadya* (a wind instrument or *suseera vadya* – Rajguru thinks it is *mukhaveena*) – was played. In another group, there were twelve *vadyakaras* to play different instruments. The person who played *khanjani* (a percussion instrument) was called *Upanga*. A flute-player was appointed, and dance and music performance was accompanied with the playing of flute. A special person was appointed for playing the *ghanta* or *tala* (large cymbals). In other words, to play a rhythm instrument. It is believed that Anangavima Deva II of Ganga dynasty had made these provisions.

The Ganga kings had married in the Chola and Chalukya royal families. As a result, there was a lot of influence of south on Orissan culture. After the Gangas, members of the Solar dynasty (Suryavansi) ruled Orissa from 1435 till 1533 AD. The Suryavansi kings were patrons of religious activities of Jagannath temple. Purosottama Deva was a *vidwan* in his own right, and he composed the *Abhinaba Gitagobinda*. One of the ministers under Prataprudra Deva, Raya Ramananda Patnaik was a great patron of arts. Although one does not find any specific document on *maharis* during this period, there is a special reference of importance in *Chaitanya Charitamruta* where the author, Krushnadas Goswami, mentions that Raya Ramananda (née Patnaik), the minister of King Prataprudra Deva during the 16th century, used to compose songs and train the *devadasis* for performances (see discussion, Devi, 1963).

During the following period, the temple was attacked several times by Muslim invaders culminating in the famous destruction and burning of the images of Lord Jagannath by Kalapahad, the Muslim General of Suleiman Karnani. Historian Abul Fazal has also documented this event (see Patnaik, p. 55). After a brief gap, Ramachandra Deva (1568-1600 AD) was crowned the king of Orissa with the help of Hindu generals of Mughal court and installed new images of Lord Jagannath. He resumed all the *sevas*. It is said that he built seven streets near the temple for the *sebayats*. One of these streets was called the *Mahari Palli* or *Anga Alasa Patna*. Apparently, there used to be six types of *maharis: Bhitara Gauni, Bahara Gauni, Nachuni, Patuari, Raja Angila* and *Gahana Mahari*. Out of these, only two – *Bhitara* and *Bahara Gauni sevas* – survived till the 1950's.

However, it is difficult to ascertain when the *parampara* stopped or if it died a natural death due to lack of patronage but several documents provide an insight into the status of the *maharis* during the period from 18th to the early part of the 20th century.

These documents also give us an idea about the confusion regarding the status of the *maharis* that prevailed during the early and later part of the 19th century. Hunter (1872) in his book "Orissa" makes some derogatory comments about the dancing girls which is refuted later by O' Malley (1908). Then there is the most important document – an article in the *Star of Utkal* (Anonymous, 1912) entitled "Deva Dasis". In addition, one finds the lists of rituals in the "Record of Rights" (1952), and lists compiled by others including that in *Karmangi* as discussed later. Since these are not only important documents but also quite inaccessible, they are presented in great detail though there is considerable overlapping between them.

Hunter (1872), in his book "Orissa", makes some interesting comments on the dancing girls in the chapter on *Jagannath*.

In page 130 of the book, he says:

> Four times every day the priests clear the sanctuary, and close the tower gates while the god is at his meals. At the door stand *Vishnuvite* ascetics, waving large fans and singing his praises. In the Pillared Hall, a choir of dancing girls enliven the idols' repast by their airy gyrations, while a few favoured servants attend him in his inner shrine.

Again in page 131 he says:

> The indecent rites that have crept into *Vishnuvism*, and which according to the spirit of the worshippers, are either high religious mysteries or simple obscenities, are represented by the Birth Festival (meaning *Janmastami*), in which the priest takes the part of the father, and dancing-girl that of the mother of Jagannath, and the ceremony of his nativity is performed to life.

Further in page 135, he states:

> Lascivious sculptures disfigure his walls, indecent ceremonies disgrace his ritual, and dancing girls with rolling eyes put the modest female worshippers to the blush.

Hence, it can be concluded that even by the end of the 19th century, the ritual had already lost its essence and spirituality. However, one of the important aspects of Hunter's reference is the fact that girls used to dance in groups four times daily. In course of time, this was perhaps reduced to solo performances during the two rituals in the early part of 1900's and then to none by 1950's.

However, one finds a more sympathetic note in the comments of O' Malley (1908) on Hunter's observations:

> The next important "*niti*" is *sakala dhupa* at which *Jagannath* is supposed to enjoy his breakfast. Meanwhile, the imaginary repast is enlivened by a girl dancing an antiquated measure to the sound of a drum.

> The chief festival is the *Chandan Yatra* which lasts for 21 days. On this occasion, Madanmohan comes forth from the temple every day and is escorted in procession to the Narendra tank. The idol is then placed on a boat and carried round the tank with music and dancing.

> Another class about whose position there has been some misconception is that of the dancing-girls (here he refers to Hunter's observations).

In refuting Hunter's observations, O' Malley says:

> It is reported that there is no indecency in any of the rites and no dancing-girl has part in the ritual. One girl, it is true, performs an antiquated dance to the accompaniment of a small drum during Jagannath's morning meal (*sakal dhupa*)

but this is not regarded as an essential part of the ceremony and her absence does not interfere with its performance. Again, at night, when all the ceremonies are over, one of the dancing-girls comes (after a bath, whatever the hour may be) and sings a song in the presence of the deity. But should any of the dancing-girls enter the inner sanctuary except on these two occasions, the whole shrine is considered defiled and *Mahasnana* or a ceremony of purifications has to be performed before the rites can continue.

Thus, in refuting Hunter's observations, O' Malley gives an idea that only two rituals were prevalent by 1908, comparable to the rituals which continued till the 1950's. However, even O' Malley gives us an insight to the fact that the rituals were mere routines and *maharis* were really not coveted.

Details of dedication of specific *maharis,* their initiation, adoption from non-Oriya families, even mortgage of the *seva* between *maharis* from temple records during the reign of Virakishore Deva (1736-1792), has been discussed by Mahapatra (1988). A document of dedication dated 1886 AD is given in the appendix 2.

Maharis who were dedicated to Lord Jagannath between 1920's to 1940's give us a glimpse into the rituals and practice before it was discontinued. The "Record of Rights" (1952) of Jagannath temple listed their name and gives us an insight into the roster duty and their wages (see Appendix 1). According to this, there were altogether nine incumbent *devadasis (Bhitara Gauni).* It is interesting to note that the name *mahari* is not used in the "Record of Rights". They are referred to as *Gaunis*, meaning singers not dancers although the details of their duties lists the dances to be performed. According to the records, out of the nine, eight (Kundamani, Kokilaprava, Taramani, Basanta, Parasamani, Binodini, Shrimati, and Subhasini) were from *Baseli Sahi* and one (Indumati) from *Markandeswara Sahi*. The services assigned to them were:

(a) To dance in *Jagamohan* during *sakala dhupa* (morning meal).
(b) Sing *Gita Govinda* after *Badasinghara* (ceremonial dressing in the evening) *bhog*.
(c) In the month of *Kartika*, sing during *bala dhupa* (early morning meal).

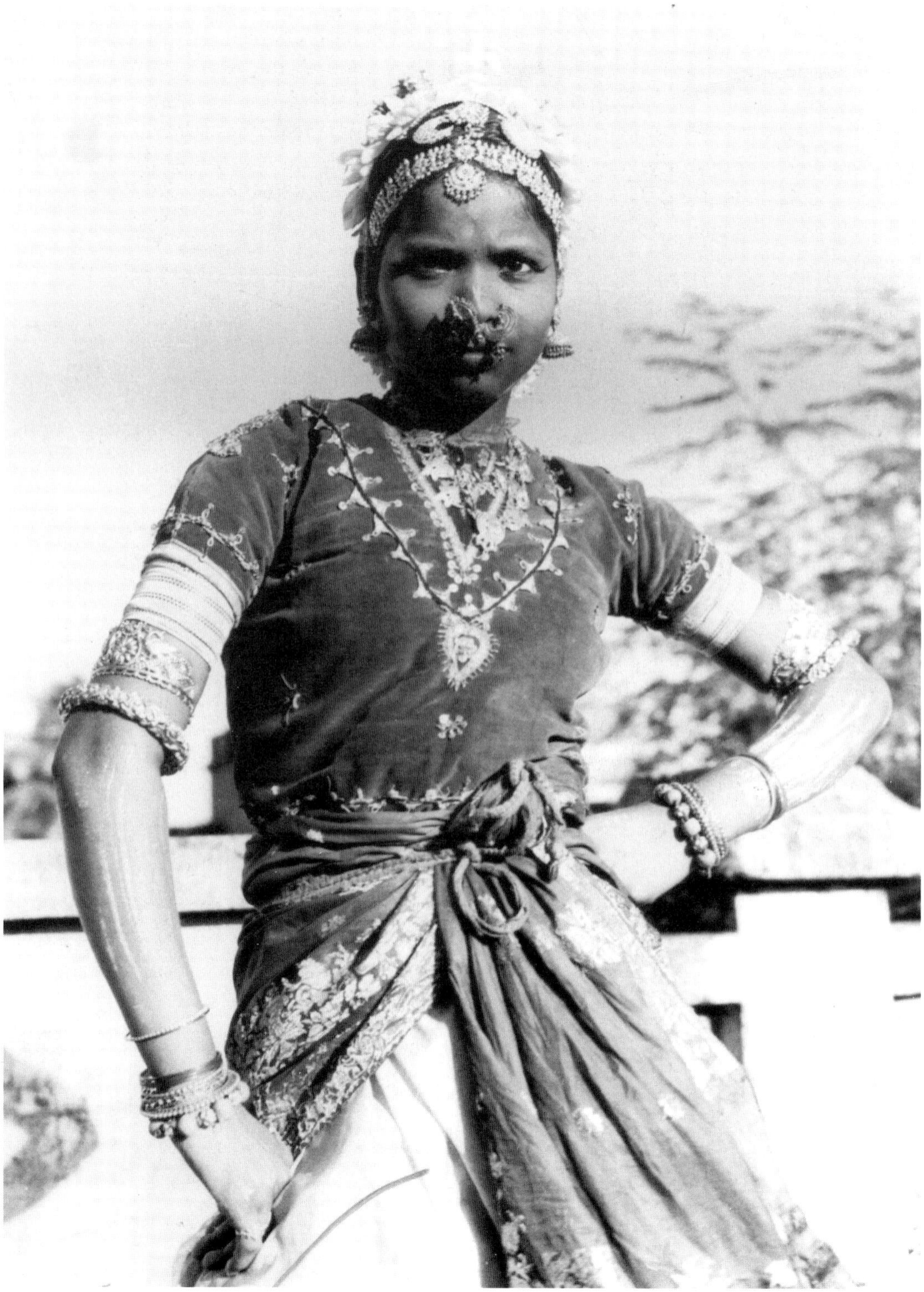

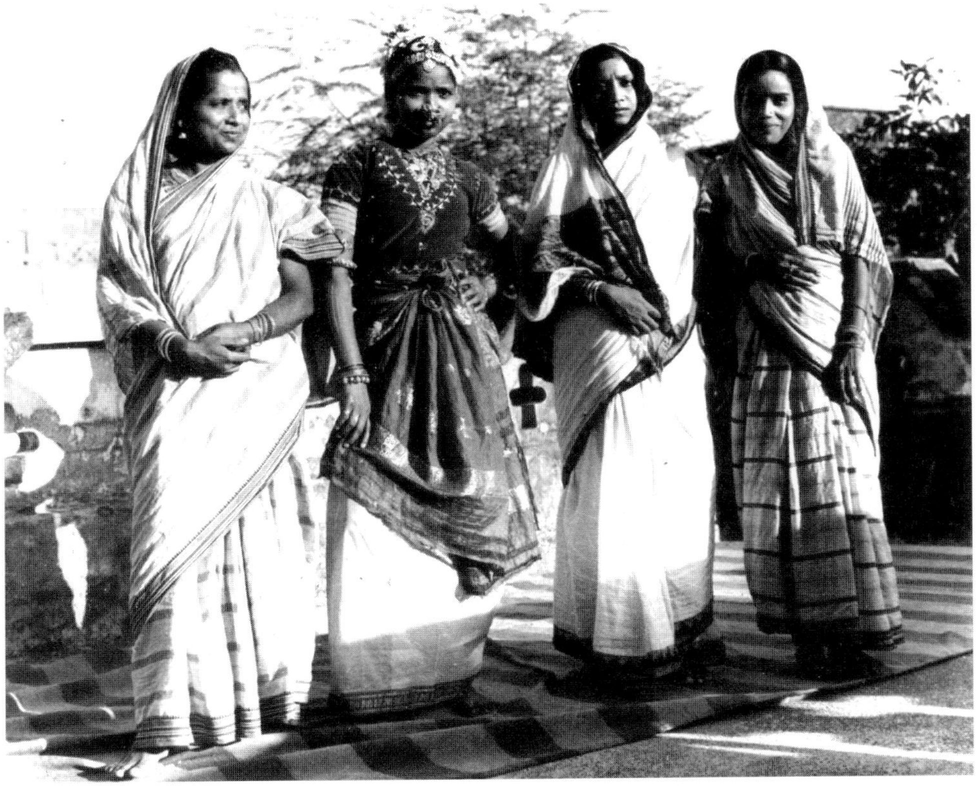

Mahari Kokilaprava, Subhasini, Haripriya and Sashiprava, 1958 (courtesy: Central Sangeet Natak Akademi, New Delhi).

(d) During the *Chandana Lagi* for 42 days during *Alata Lagi* (fanning), they will sing in *Anasara pindi.*

(e) For 42 days during *Chandana Lagi*, they will dance in *Jagamohan.*

(f) Dance in Madanmohan's *Chapa* (boating) for 21 days.

(g) Sing (*Mangala gana*) in *Rukmini Vivaha* in the Lakshmi temple.

(h) On the day of *Niladri Vijé* they will accompany Lakshmi to the *Veta mandap* (meeting pendal) and participate in the "Mock fight dialogue" on behalf of Lakshmi; they will dance in the *Gundicha mandap* on the first day.

(i) In the month of *Aswina*, in the *puja* called *Shola-puja* (special *puja* for 16 days in the temple of Bimala) they would go in procession. During the closing ceremonies (*Pahuda majana*) of Bimala temple they will sing *Malashri* (lyrics dedicated to *Devis*). For these 16 days only, the *devadasis* (and not other ladies) are allowed inside the Bimala temple.

FACING PAGE : *Mahari Subhasini, 1958 (courtesy: Central Sangeet Natak Adademi, New Delhi).*

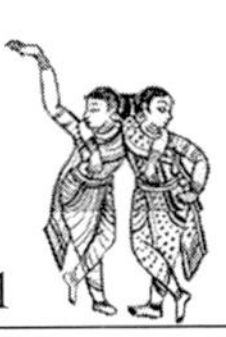

(j) In the palace, they will go in procession during *Kanaka Durga puja.*
(k) On the day of *Pusyaviseka*, they will go with *Mudirastha* for *arti* to his house.
(l) In the month of *Phalguna*, *Phagu-dasami* onwards, they will participate in the rituals in the *Vedi* (*Pandal*) during *bhoga*. On *Chaturdasi*, they will play *phagu* (holi) in the *Jagamohan* of *Lakshmi* temple with *Mudirastha.*
(m) During *Naba patrika*, they will participate in the ritual for goddess Durga in the palace.
(n) They will dance in the *Snana Vedi* (*Pandal* for ceremonial bath).
(o) During *Nabakalevara*, they will do *Hulahuli* (an auspicious sound produced by the movement of the tongue) as they accompany the *daru* (sacred log).

The "Record of Rights", lays down the turn or roster *(bedhas)* in which the *devadasis* had to do the ritual and their payments in terms of food (local cakes). The same "Record of rights" further states that the dates which have not been assigned to the *devadasis*, the two *Sampradaya nijogas* will do the ritual on alternate years. All the *devadasis* were entitled to *Vaishnabagni* (at the time of the funeral ceremony, the fire to light the pyre comes from the eternal flame from Jagannath temple).

It also states the gratifications for becoming a *devadasi.* The *devadasis* have to be initiated which is referred to as *Saribandha.* They cannot marry or lead an unholy life. If they violate these rules, the ritual will be discontinued. They can adopt girls from *Pani sparsa jati* (not lower caste). They will be eligible for *Saribandha* or initiation only after being proficient in singing and dancing. If they have any difficulty in sticking to their schedule, they may appoint the "*Samprada* for dance" to do the ritual but not of any other category. It is believed that *Samprada* refers to Telegu *devadasis.* According to Rajguru (1978), *Telegu Sampradaya* was entitled to singing *Gita Govinda* during Prataprudra Deva's time.

It further states that in older times, the *devadasis* were assigned 18 *bati* land but it was not so during the 1950's. However, the reason for the discontinuity is not known. They also used to receive Rs. 9/- (Rupees nine only) for their *Habisa* (a restricted vegetarian diet) expenses. This is because on the day of dance the *devadasis* used to be on a *habisa* diet.

In addition to the "Record of Rights", the *sevas* (rituals) of the Jagannath temple have been compiled by several people, out of which the report by Puri Collector Grome, Pandit Suryanarayan Das' book "The Jagannath Mandir" and "Karmangi" are important. All these have been compiled by Mohanty (1985). Although, discussing them in detail may sound repetitive, they are discussed in detail here as most of these materials as mentioned earlier are important and not readily available for reference.

Collector Grome's list contains the rituals of *Binakara* (no. 134), *Samprada nijoga* (no. 200) and *Nartaki nijoga* (no. 201). In the list of Pandit Suryanarayan Das' one finds *Binakara* (no. 20), *Bhitara gayani* (no. 21), *Samprada nijoga* (no. 22), *Madeli* (no. 23) and *Gita Govinda* (no. 28). Perhaps the most important is the "Karmangi" which has been edited by Mohanty (1958), who opines that some of the descriptions fit into the 16th century. In any case, "Karmangi" gives details of the *sevas* out of which the following are relevant here.

Upangiya: The *sevaka* who will supervise the ritual with *Mina nahaka* and *Mahari*, etc.

Mahariė: The one with *baharonijoga* should not cross *Jaya vijaya dwara. Bhitara gauni palia* should go up to *Kalaghata dwara* (the last door leading to the *Ratnabedi* or sanctum sanctorum), should recite *Mangalagana* in marriages, and go in the *Guali patuar* (procession) on *Champak dwadasi*. During *ratha* (meaning *Ratha jatra*), during the *Bahuda* (return car festival) of *Parameswara* (meaning Jagannath), should go in the *patuar* of *Parama Lakshmi*. Wherever *Mahalakshmi* goes, they will accompany, reciting the *Mangala*. Daily, during the *Pahada* (retirement of Jagannath every night), they will sing near the *Kalaghata dwara*. Everyday during *dhupa* (meal), they will perform *Alasha dance* in front of *Garuda* (meaning *Garuda sthambha*). They will dance daily in *Mahapravu's Chapa* (Lord's boat). They should not have physical contact with others. When *sevakas* leave, they should bow but they should not bow down before others. During *Nanda Utsav*, two of them should act as *Rohini* and *Yasoda*.

They should go in procession. During the *Bahudabije'* (return car festival), they should take part in a dialogue (perhaps meaning the dialogue of Lakshmi with Lord Jagannath as she takes exception to the fact that Lord Jagannath does not take her out with him during the car festival. Therefore, she gives him a hard time before letting him in – a rather human touch in the ritual). They should recite *Mangala* in the *Utsavs* (celebrations) in the house of the *sevaka* and perform their duty in the king's palace who is comparable to *Parameswar*. The duty ends with the words *Bije' abara tulaibe*, meaning any other duties in the procession of Lord (Bije').

P 36 - ***Madeli Khatani Nijoga***: *Mina nahaka khatani sevaka*. During the procession of the Lord, he will play the *Madala* in the middle between the *Kanshari* and *Ghantua*. During the *dhupa seva*, and during the *Chapa*, he will play with *Bahara gauni*. During the procession of Ramachandra *(Ramachandraka Bimana bijé)*, he will play *Malashri* (in the modern day context, *Malashri* are specific songs sung in peculiar style in praise of goddesses).

P 47 - **Binakara:** His *seva* is *Narada seva*. During the *Pahada* (closure of the door to *sanctum sanctorum)*, time will play the *Bina* and sing *Kalasha* (in the modern day context, *Kalasha* is a melodic simplistic pattern of *Chhanda* style of singing. For example, *Dandare shuvila Rama Krushna beni bhai* tune) near the *Kalaghata dwara*. Just before *Pahada* the *gauni* will sing *Gita Govinda*.

In addition, the following is the most informative document on *devadasis* of Orissa. Because it gives an insight into the whole system at a critical period, I would like to quote the whole article from Star of Utkal (Anonymous, 1912).

The spirit of the article indicates that the *devadasi* system was already under social and economical stress leading to moral problems. The author (anonymous), obviously sympathetic to their problems, compares them to the nuns and gives suggestions to improve the system. Further in the article, the *maharis* are referred to as *Mairis* with an interesting interpretation.

DEVA DASIS

In this much married age, if we may get a band of noble Hindu girls devoted to the service of God and man, what harm? Married to Jagannath, the Lord of the Universe, she is the mother of his children, bound to serve God, her husband, bound to look after his children. In Oriya language, she is called "Ma-iri," or

Matri or Mother, the same name that nuns had, Nun coming from the Pali word "Nani" and "Matri" in Sanskrit. If enrollment to nunship is not stopped, why should enrollment to Mairiship be? Many things were alleged against nuns, as many things are against Mairis. What more devoted band of workers, servants of God, these handmaids, are found in the World, in trouble and calamity, in the sick room, in war-field, in fire, famine and cyclone than the Nun ? If the Deva Dasi has deteriorated, bring her under control, put a Mataji, as a Mother Superior, an abbess, over her to educate and train her up to devote herself to the service of God and man. Such Mother Superiors are not rare, the Mahakali Pathasalas have shown. The Deva Dasi lived on bequests left by the old Rajas of Orissa; still they get honour and allowance; so it is not difficult to bring them under control. Their number is not large. According to calculations made by the government, there are only 100 in Puri but the number is not more than fifty, and besides Puri there is none anywhere also in Aryavarta or between the Himalayas and the Vindhya hills. The Deva Dasis of Jagannath are not like the Dwarees of Southern India, that go through mock marriages to live a life of prostitution. To abolish the class of Deva Dasis would not only be interfering with Hindu religion, it would be ruining an institution that may be turned to very useful purposes.

The institution may not have any Shastric sanction, but it has a hoary antiquity to its existence. The Deva Dasis of Orissa are the chronological successors of the Budhistic Sthaviras or Theras, whose Gathas or religious songs in Pali recently been translated into English by Mrs. Rhys Devids and has charmed the Western world. On the jambs at the Jaya vijaya door of the Audience Hall, amongst several inscriptions, we read (thirty-two years ago from Dr. Rajendra Lal's Antiquities of Orissa), an inscription by Maharaja Pratap Rudra Dev ordering the singing of Gita Govinda by Deva Dasis before Jagannath every evening from "Sanjha Dhupa to Bara Singhar". Pratap Rudra was a contemporary of Sri Chaitanya. A gentleman brought his daughter, as mentioned in the Chaitanya Mangal, to marry Chaitanya. However, being an ascetic he could not accept the girl, so she was married to Jagannath. The author of Gita Govinda, Sri Jaya Deva Goswami, married Padma Vati who was intended for Jagannath. So we find the custom of dedicating girls to Jagannath obtained at Puri for a thousand years.

There is no dedication of girls nowadays by pilgrims or outsiders. The custom is now confined amongst a few families, who are held in special honour for their connection with the temple. Sri Krishna's Gopinees are Jagannath's Mairees, companions, maids, and co-wives of Lakshmi. Mairees are of two classes; the superior class are allowed to enter the inner shrine, help in temple service, dance and sing before the God. The lower class help in menial work in the morning hours. They may sing and dance, but are not allowed to enter the inner shrine. The two classes have special privileges, allowances and prerequisites.

The Mairee Families marry. To keep the connection with the one or two girls are devoted to temple service. On reaching puberty, they apply to Raja – the Temple Manager – to be recognised as Mairee. On proof of age and previous good conduct, a saree is given to them in recognition and their names are registered. A Mairee is not allowed to marry, to leave the precincts of Puri and go out at night time, except to the temple premises. They are known to the pilgrims as Kumarees or maidens. Not more than two Mairees on an average are recruited in a year.

No doubt many Mairees fall. In all countries, poverty leads to immorality. Unlike other professions, an inexperienced apprentice in harlotry earns more than the experienced ones. If sufficient allowance may be provided from the temple and the Parichha be compelled to exercise strict supervision and if proper arrangements be made for education, the Mairees may be made into a very useful body of helpers. They cannot be turned out of the temple, but they may be considerably improved.

(Anonymous, 1912)

Thus by 1912, the *devadasis* were known as *mairiees* and a clear class structure was prevalent. The *Bhitar Gaunis* conducting rituals within the *sanctum sanctorum,* had a superior status than the *Bahara Gaunis* conducting rituals outside the *sanctum sanctorum.*

Some of the procedures mentioned in this article underwent changes during the latter period. According to the present-day *maharis,* they came from two sources. One, of course, is the hereditary line as mentioned in the article, the other was by adoption from *Pani sparsa jati.* Earlier, on reaching puberty only, the girl was eligible for being recruited as a *mahari.* But the present-day *maharis* were initiated between ages 5 to 10 (before reaching puberty stage). Taramani, Chandamani and Harapriya were initiated under Raja Mukunda Deva and the rest under Ramachandra Deva. Apparently, due to lack of patronage and deterioration of the system, there was a shortage of girls in the older age group, hence in order to carry on the tradition the families resorted to what can best be described as "Child marriage with Lord Jagannath." In order to be initiated into the system, their families had to deposit Rs. 20/- to Rs. 30/-, which was quite a large sum of money in the early part of 20th century. After obtaining the approval for the initiation, the services of the *Charchika* (who applies the sandalwood paste on them), the *Maluni* (lady supplying flowers) and the *Pujaka* (priest) were requisitioned. On the day of the marriage, she was bedecked with jewellery, flowers and sandalwood paste like a typical Oriya bride. During the evening *puja* ceremony, Patjoshi Mahapatra, who was the official representative of Puri Raja, conducted an elaborate marriage ceremony before Lord Jagannath. At the end of the marriage ceremony, Patjoshi Mahapatra took a piece of silk cloth from Lord Jagannath and tied it on the head of his new bride. This ceremony is referred to as the *Saribandha* reminiscent of the *saree* of yesteryears. In the 18th century, *sarees* were from the wardrobes of goddesses in the temple (Mahapatra, 1988).

After the *Saribandha*, Patjoshi Mahapatra used to put rice, betel nut and flowers in the hands of the bride, who walked around the temple (*Parikrama*) and then walked back to her house in a procession and offered the rice, betel nut and flowers into the *Kani* (*anchal* of the *saree*) of her mother – a mark signifying her marriage, went to the house *Chaura* (the abode of goddess Brindabati which is essentially a platform which houses the *Tulasi* plant – a regular feature in houses in Orissa) and then the final *puja* was performed. The marriage typically ended with a sumptuous feast.

One interesting aspect of the genealogy of a *mahari* is that since according to the tradition it is a purely mother-to-daughter system in which the mother is essentially a virgin, both the real mother and father of a *mahari* become insignificant. In this *amaternate* and *apaternate* system, in order to be inducted as a *mahari*, an adoption is a must. Apparently, there was a two-tier vigilance system of the temple management to ensure that the *maharis* led a proper life. Out of these two, the *Mina Nahaka* was in-charge of bringing them to the temple and their safe return after the completion of the ritual. The *Sahi Nahaka* or *Sahinahaka* (*Sahi* meaning the particular area in which they reside) was to supervise that they led a pious and proper life. Since *devadasis* lived in different areas of Puri, there were *Sahi Nahakas* allotted for each area. Later, Kokilaprava lived in *Betra gali* (lane) of *Markanda sahi*, Indumati in *Markandeswar sahi*, Chandamani in *Hadagadin gali* and Harapriya (née *Dunguri*) in *Kundhei benta sahi* in their own residences. Sashimani lives in a rented house. Late *mahari* Haripriya explained that because she was an *Apartiani* (meaning that the child born before her died), her parents gave her an insignificant nickname *Dunguri* (a practice still prevalent in Orissa where it is believed that an insignificant name will ward off the evil eye which led to the death of the child born earlier).

Coming to the rituals performed by these *maharis,* there were the two daily rituals, one during the *sakala dhupa* (morning meal of Lord Jagannath), with the *Jaya Vijaya Dwara* (door to sanctum sanctorum) closed. On the day the *mahari* had her turn (*Pali*), she had to sanctify herself with a ritual bath and dress in her finest *saree* bedecked with jewellery and decorated with *chandan* (sandalwood paste). She used to wear her *saree* with a *Kania Kachha,* a style of wrapping unique, to *maharis*, from waist down. She wore a specially decorated velvet blouse called *kanchala.* She used to go in a procession led by the *Mina Nahaka*, had a thick veil on, and used to walk bare foot the whole distance from her house to the temple with her eyes focussed on the ground. She was not to look or converse with any man either on her way to the temple or while dancing. (Late *Singhari* Shyama Sunder Kar who gave me the first lessons in Odissi dance, used to insist that I apply *chandan* on my face and arms just like *maharis.* It consisted of dipping the finger in a bowl of *chandan* paste, and drawing stripes on the cheeks, forehead and arms. When I enquired about what at that time appeared to be amusing to decorate one's body, *Kabichandra* Kalicharan Patnaik told me that the *chandan* was used as a repellant for the flies. It was considered inauspicious to have a fly sit on a *mahari* during her procession to the temple for her ritual).

In the temple, the *mahari* used to dance in front of the *Garuda Sthamba* in the *Natamandira*, facing the *Jaya Vijaya Dwara.* On reaching the *Natamandira* she used to take off the veil, tie it at her waist like a *natabari* and dance to the accompaniment of *mardala*. The *mardala* player (exclusively men) used to come from traditional *madeli* families. The dance started as soon as the *Jaya Vijaya Dwara* closed for offering of morning meal (*sakala dhupa*), with the *Parichha* presiding with his gold cane. The dance lasted till the *Jaya Vijaya Dwara* opened. The time period varied from day to day. The dance consisted of simplistic movements to the chanting of *bols* (*ukutas*) by the *madeli*. The dance was performed in a cyclical pattern going over and over the same piece which assured a continuous performance for the uncertain time period. When after my first performance in the Youth Festival in 1954, Mohan Khokar came to Orissa to get a first hand knowledge of this style of dance, he could arrange for only one *mahari* (Kokilaprava*)* to show the dance. I quote Shri Khokar (1985) as he is perhaps the only outsider to see a *Mahari* dress up to perform (though outside the temple), in the 1950's, along with late *Kabichandra* Kalicharan Patnaik.

> Kali babu had managed to get himself and me invited to lunch with the Raja of Puri at his palace, and thrown into the bargain was a dance by a *mahari*. The *mahari* was Kokilaprava. Her dance was a big letdown. Attired garishly, overdecked with silver, she did go through her paces, but clumsily, and with no feeling. Nothing registered. I felt hollow within, cheated, and a surge of pity for the artiste, and the art, overtook me. My recklessness, of course. *Maharis* had long since stopped dancing, and seeing but one of them was surely no way to gauge the worth of the art.

According to the *maharis*, the same pieces of dance were taught by the adopted mother to daughter and practiced with the *madeli* at their homes. The dancers who initially belonged to a separate category called *Bahara Gauni*, did not perform the evening ritual which was done by the other category, the *Bhitara Gauni*. But according to the present *maharis*, all of them performed as *Bahara Gauni* until they reached puberty and then they switched their ritual to *Bhitara Gauni*. Obviously, due to shortage of girls for this ritual, the two distinct categories of earlier years had merged into one.

The second daily ritual by *Bhitara Gauni*, literally meaning "inside singer", was in the evening and was restricted to singing only. Sometimes they sang *astapadis* from the *Gita Govinda* but mostly Oriya *jananas* (*bhajans*) with gesticulation (not *hastabhinaya)*. The songs, even *astapadis* of *Jayadeva*, were sung in simplistic melodic patterns, and at times they only recited the songs. Just as complex dance patterns are not essential for service to God, complex musical patterns are not necessary for the service either. What is important in ritualistic practice of dance and music is the spirit in which it is performed.

No one knows when exactly these rituals came to extinction although different people give different dates. But by 1954, the ritual had stopped completely. Only the *Bhitara Gauni* ritual was revived in the 1960's and *mahari* Kokilaprava resumed her duties until her death.

In the present-day context, in spite of the views of Hunter (1872), the *maharis* used to be accepted as very auspicious women, as being wives of Lord Jagannath they never became widows (called *ahia* in Oriya). They were coveted for singing songs (*mangala gana*) during the *Brataupanayana* (thread ceremony) and marriage ceremonies held at Puri (*maharis* were not allowed to go outside the border of Puri). Late Mrs. Bhagabati Panigrahi once told me that *mahari* Harapriya sang at her marriage cermony held in Puri, in the 1930's. Although the *maharis* claim to have danced in Madanamohana's *chapa* (boat) during *Chandan Jatra*, as I have said earlier, by 1955, at least it had stopped completely. (Personally I had gone to see it but was disappointed to learn that the ritual had been discontinued.)

SAMPRADA NIJOGA AND OTHER *SEVAS* PERTAINING TO MUSIC

A class named *Samprada nijoga* refers to dancing girls who dance at the time of *Patuara* (procession) in the *Chatisa nijoga* (thirty-six categories of services employed in the temple, Mishra, 1971). As mentioned earlier, they are believed to be descendants of a group of dancers and musicians brought in from the South by Choraganga Deva. Thus, initially *Samprada nijoga* had peripheral duties but the "Record of Rights" (Appendix 1) mentions that they can substitute for *mahari* duty, indicative of the subsequent acceptance of *Samprada nijoga* for duties inside the temple perhaps due to the shortage of *maharis*.

One more *nijoga* which is of prime importance in the context of rituals of music and dance in Jagannath temple is *Gita Govinda seva* for reciting the *Gita Govinda* before the Lord at *Chandan Lagi.* What is interesting is that although most of the *nijogas* are through hereditary lines, some of the services are open to public who could apply and be granted the permission for this service. *Gita Govinda seva* and *Chamar seva* (waving the fly whisk) are the two belonging to these categories. Late *Kabichandra* Kalicharan Patnaik had been granted the *Chamar seva*; implicit in being indoctrinated to this *seva* means that at death they are entitled to *Vaishnabagni* (the fire from the *eternal flame* in the Jagannath temple for lighting their funeral pyre).

To conclude, if one has to be objective about the status of *maharis,* I would think that a sequence of glory, degeneration, near-extinction and recuperation will be most appropriate. Glory period was marked by establishment of the ritual, codification of the ritual and lavish grants to *maharis* for a comfortable life in appreciation of their life-long dedication and voluntary "unmarried status" for all practical purposes. Here marriage to Lord Jagannath was more at mental than physical level. During the degeneration period, the morals were low, the support scanty and considerable exploitation due to their vulnerability. Recruitment was probably discontinued in the late 40's because after this period, no new *mahari* was initiated. The recuperation in status (though not in ritual) is intimately related to the revival of Odissi dance. With the interest in the tradition of Odissi dance both in Orissa as well as from outside Orissa, a lot of interest has been generated in the *mahari* system. From 1950 onwards, the few living *maharis* who were sometimes referred to in derogatory terms like *daris* (prostitutes) in Puri, became more and more confident and fought for their rights as practitioners of music and dance. Finally, Kokilaprava went back to the ritual. Almost all of them received pensions as retired artistes from Orissa Government. One interesting point should be made here that *maharis* probably lost their social status in Puri but have been and still are revered by pilgrims visiting the Puri temple. I was told by Late Dr. Mayadhar Mansinha that once when he was in the Jagannath temple (perhaps in the late 30's or early 40's), there was a lot of commotion, everyone running to the *Natamandira.* By the time he reached it, he found a dancer completing her dance and leaving with the *Madeli.* The pilgrims rolled on the ground in ecstacy as it was considered to be very auspicious to roll on the floor and be coated with the dust off the *mahari's* feet. It has been said that there was immense excitement when Kokilaprava came to sing before the Lord at night.

THE GOTIPUAS

An event immensely significant for the evolution of Odissi dance was the establishment of *gotipua* system where boys of tender age were trained in the art of dancing and singing like *maharis* and started performing for general public. They were of course not allowed to dance inside the temple but eventually participated in many ritualistic festivals connected with Lord Jagannath.

Goti in Oriya means "single" and *pua* means a "boy". In the absence of any historical document, speculations abound about the origin of this system. Out of these, only the leading views will be discussed here. According to Panigrahi (1960):

> the Gotipua dance appears to have originated in the reign of Pratapa Rudradeva (1497-1540 AD) and gained popularity in the subsequent Muslim Period on account of the rigidity of the *purdha* system which led to the seclusion of women and made their presence scarce on festive occasions.

Many favour the view that Ramananda Ray, the minister of Pratapa Rudra Deva née Prataprudra Deva who was a devout *Vaishnavite* and an expert in music and dance, probably encouraged worship according to *Sakhi Bhava* and introduced the custom of the temple dances being performed by boys dressed as girls and not by women as was the custom elsewhere (Kothari, 1965). But there is no mention of this in the *Chaitanya Charitamruta* which has mentioned about Ramananda teaching *abhinaya* to *maharis.*

But an interesting view is encountered in the introduction to *Kabisurya Granthabali* and *Jibanacharita* by Gopal Chandra Praharaj (1928). These are perhaps the best documents so far as the *gotipua* system is concerned.

Shri Praharaj writes that *Kishore Chandranana Champu* (popularly called *Kishori Champu*) is well-known throughout Orissa. The *gotipua* troupes who cannot sing the *Kishori Champu* in appropriate *ragaragini* and *parija* (*mudras*) are not liked by the public. He further states that after the *Chhanda* (a style of singing in *sthai* only without any *antara)* period of Upendra Bhanja, Gopala Krushna, Banamali, etc. appeared and composed Odissi music. At that time, Ganjam was in Madras (now Chennai) and the music was influenced considerably by the Telegu people from Andhra. Further, in the music and dance performances the vulgar dance by prostitutes used to be prevalent. According to Praharaj, Oriyas created *gotipua* troupes as an alternative to the vulgar dance of the Andhra prostitutes.

An interesting definition of *gotipua* appears in the *Purnachandra Oriya Bhashakosha*, Part II (1932) and IV (1934), compiled by Gopal Chandra Praharaj. According to him, in the *Sangita dala* (music groups), one boy sings and dances. In *Utkala*, tender-aged good looking boys are dressed as girls who sing, dance and do *abhinaya* on *Pouranika* (mythology) themes. If these *Pouranika abhinetas* are more than one, they are known as *Sakhipila*. The boy who sings while dancing is called *gotipua*. *Gotipuas* also exhibit some extremely difficult *Bandha* (acrobatics) or *Bayam* (exercises). The *Natapilas* dance and sing; and by *angabhangis* and hand movement *(karadees)*, express the meaning of the songs.

Whatever the origin may be, the Odissi dance field has been dominated by the *gotipua* system. At the turn of the century, *gotipua* troupes were patronised all over Orissa. Even my own (Priyambada's) paternal grand-father, Late Shri Jagabandhu Mohanty, who was a *zamindar* (landlord) in Apsarapur (Gopalpur), in Jajpur (formerly Cuttack) district, used to patronise a troupe. If *mahari* tradition was the source of Odissi dance, the *gotipua* system sustained and developed it. It is no coincidence that all the leading *gurus* today were trained as *gotipuas* under some legendary *gurus* like Late Shri Mohan Mahapatra and Late Shri Chandrasekhar Patnaik, etc. As Praharaj writes, literature was intertwined to *gotipua* dance:

> the *gurus* had to be well-versed in literature to interpret the lyrics of the songs that were danced away.

In my opinion, *abhinaya* developed in the repertoire during the period when *gotipuas* started interpreting the meaning of the songs of Kabisurya, Banamali and Gopalkrushna. Whatever the *maharis* sang as a ritual during the *Badasinghara Vesha* was more of a gesticulation than *abhinaya*. Mention

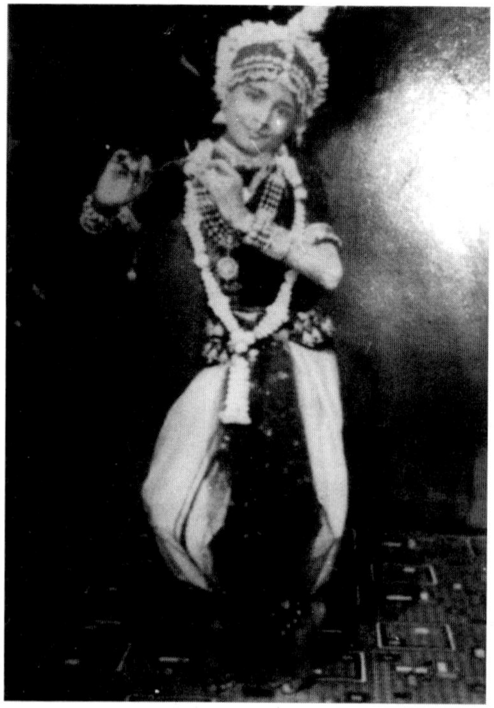

Gotipua (Akhada Pila) attached to Jagannath Temple, 1967 (courtesy: Rabinarayan Panda).

may be made that Raya Ramananda taught two *maharis* how to interpret the meaning of the songs and made them perform in front of Lord Jagannath according to the text of *Chaitanya Charitamruta* – the only reference to *abhinaya* by *maharis*. We do not even have a legend what to speak of document of any *Mahari* being skilled in *abhinaya*. Even the *maharis* who used to sing at *Badasinghara Vesha* were called *Bhitara Gaunis* (meaning "inside singers"), the emphasis being more on singing than *abhinaya*. No wonder in the fading years of *maharis*, at least one *mahari*, Parasamani, could even become a singer in the All India Radio, Cuttack.

However, one of the important contribution of *gotipua* system was the spread of devotional songs based on Radha-Krishna throughout Orissa. People were constantly subjected to the lyrics of great Oriya poets by the *gotipua* troupes – no less a feat for spreading and popularising of literature in Orissa. Whatever the origin may be, the dance became so popular that it could be absorbed into rituals in some temples as well. During *Chandan Jatra*, a *gotipua* (also called *akhadapila*) used to dance in the *chapa* (boat) of Shri Ramakrushna. In 1955, I myself witnessed a *gotipua* of very tender age being carried on his father's shoulders after the *chapa*. The little boy was so exhausted that he was asleep. Apparently, by 1955, it was just a symbolic ritual that the boy was dressed and went in the boat but did not dance. But an interesting aspect about the dance in *chapa* came up during my discussions with the *maharis*. They mentioned that a girl of a *Mahari* family, Binodini, was so skilled in dancing (meaning pure dance), that she could impersonate a *gotipua* and travel in the *chapa* of Ramakrushna. This indicated the difference between the performance of a *mahari* as opposed to that of a *gotipua* in the *chapa* of Ramakrushna. Obviously, it was an issue of honour for a dancer to perform in the moving *chapa* of Ramakrushna. The other one was mostly restricted to less vigorous dance of the *maharis* in the *chapa* of Madanamohana. The *mahari* also used to sing in the *chapa*. One such song is by Banamali (*Dine na Dakibu Radhika boli*) sung in a traditional tune which I used for my *abhinaya* in early the 1960's and which

FACING PAGE : *Present day Gotipua (courtesy: Central Sangeet Natak Akademi, New Delhi).*

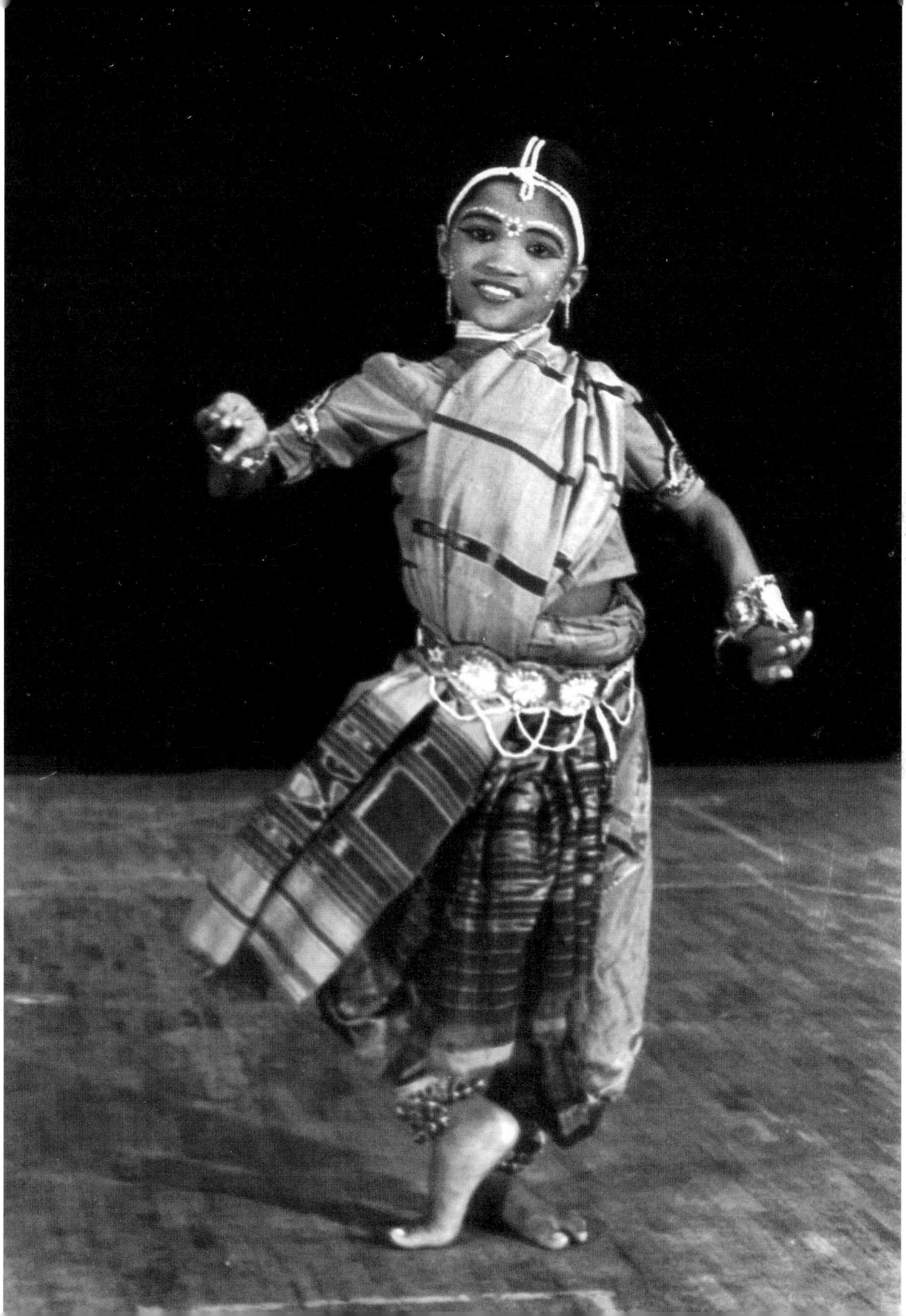

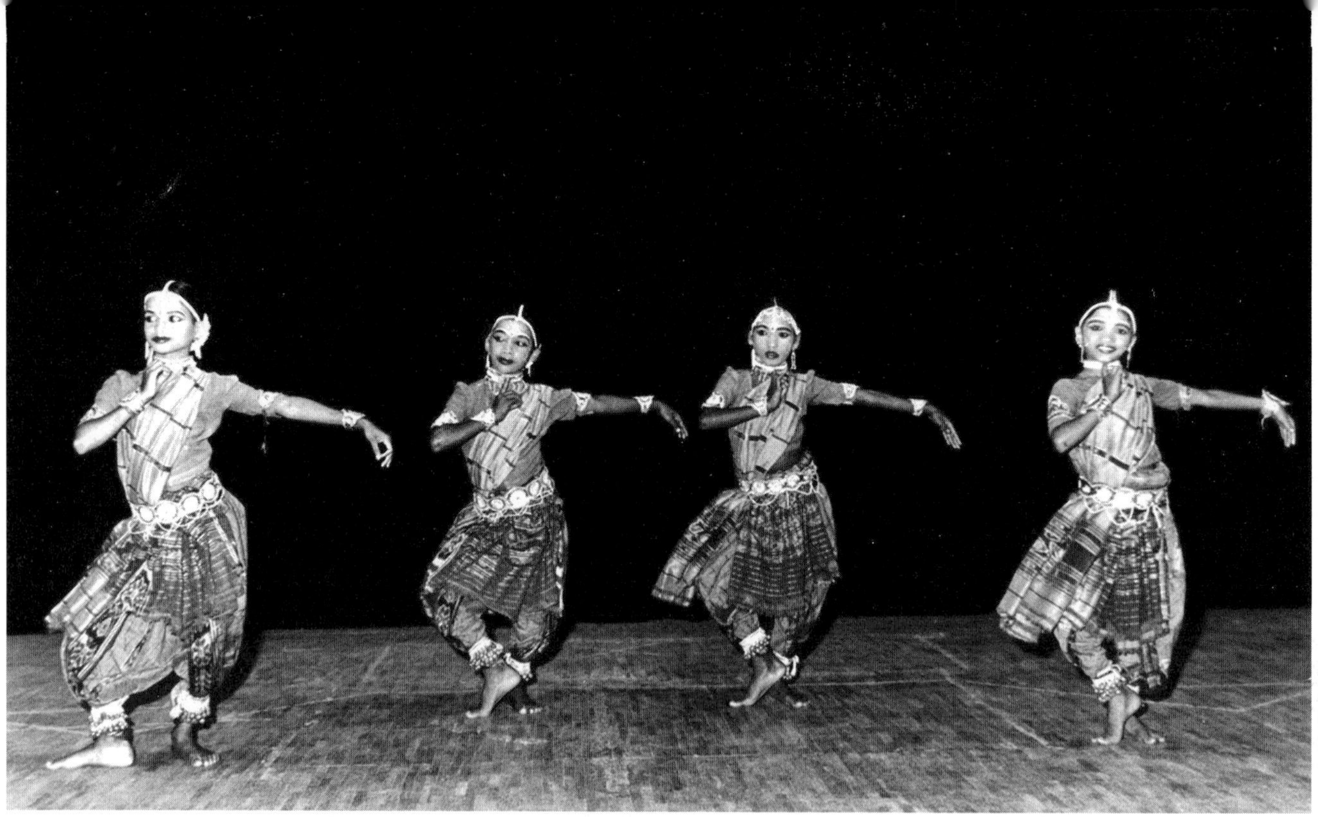

Gotipuas in group (courtesy: Central Sangeet Natak Akademi, New Delhi).

remains a popular piece till today. On the occasion of certain religious festivals, namely *Chandan Jatra* and *Jhoolan Jatra*, *gotipuas* still perform. During *Jhoolan Jatra*, most of the well-known *gotipua* troupes of the state assemble at Puri and perform in different *maths* even today. But the dance itself is degenerated, the lyrics in disarray – a rather sad affair in general.

It has been mentioned in the *Madala Panji* that during the 17th century, Gajapati Shri Ramachandra Deva established *Satasahi Akhada* (*Akhada* meaning gymnasium, in seven places). These were centres for exercises as well as for training in music and *gotipua* dance. This system spread to different villages in Orissa so that many villages, specially in Puri and Cuttack districts, had their own *akhadas* – a sort of cultural centre so to say. The *gotipua* system flourished in the 18th and 19th centuries when they took to interpreting lyrics of *Vaishnavite* poets for *abhinaya* as mentioned earlier. Although Jayadeva wrote his *Gita Govinda* in the 12th century, there is no mention of *abhinaya* to *Gita Govinda* either by the *maharis* or the *gotipuas*. In our opinion, it was during the influence and immense popularity of the Oriya poems by *Vaishnavite* poets that *abhinaya* became an integral part of dance. *Abhinaya* to *Gita*

Govinda has been of more recent origin in Odissi dance, inspired through the *Jayadeva* drama produced by Orissa theatres of Late *Kabichandra* Kalicharan Patnaik and incorporated into dance, gradually reaching a peak during the revival period of Odissi during 1950's to 1960's. As mentioned earlier, *maharis* only used to sing *Gita Govinda* without any *abhinaya* during their *seva*.

One of the major difference between the *mahari* and *gotipua* dance was that *gotipuas* sang while dancing – *bachika abhinaya* in the true sense. while, the *maharis* either sang or danced but they never sang while dancing.

The accompanying musical instruments for *gotipua nrutya* was *mardala* and *gini*. The *guru* used to chant the *ukutas* (*bols*) and conduct the dance. Usually, *gotipuas* used to stand with folded hands while a *sloka* devoted to *Ganapati* was sung. Then they used to start singing, punctuating the singing with spurts of pure dance. Generally, the *gotipua* used to sing a line and provide interpretations in several ways while the line used to be repeated by the *guru* and the *palias* (singers who used to provide vocal support as and when necessary). The *mardala* used to be smaller than the *mardala (pakhawaj)* that is being used in modern day Odissi dance. The *mardala* player used to hang the *mardala* at his waist level and play in standing position. Later, on other instruments like violin, etc. were used.

During the 19th century and the early part of the 20th century, *gotipua* system was influenced by the *Sakhi nacha*, also called *Dakhini nrutya*, from the South. Even the *saree* was wrapped in the *dakhini* style by *gotipuas* during the 40's and 50's. Under the influence of *Sakhi nacha* the *Bhakti bhava*, in *gotipua* dance was gradually replaced with *Sringara rasa*. Instead of a literary and intellectual exercise, the boys were trained to entice the rich clientele by vulgar interpretations and suggestive movements. But in spite of the degeneration, whatever was left with the *gotipua gurus* and *gotipuas* provided enough material for the reconstruction of Odissi dance after Priyambada's performance in 1954 in the First Inter-University Youth Festival at Talkatora garden, New Delhi.

At present, *gotipuas* are being trained in a few villages, specially in Cuttack and Puri districts. An attempt is being made to nourish and revive the whole system. The first "*gotipua* meet" was held a few years back to provide impetus for the revival of the system. But it was obvious that the modern day *gotipuas* have not only been influenced by the modern day Odissi, a sort of reverse pattern from 1950's, but also gone are the *gurus* who used to be well-versed in the lyrics of the songs that were danced away. The songs they sing now is often wrong – the gyrations lack the finesse due to lack of proper training. The emphasis is more on acrobatics than interpretation of lyrics. It may be of interest as an endangered ancestor of Odissi dance but has very little relevance to the modern day Odissi dance. Odissi is much more sophisticated in terms of music, movements and costume. But, from my personal experience, I have been much more inspired by the *gotipuas* of 40's and 50's because there was spark in both singing and the dance. I myself (Priyambada) learnt a lot of the movements by watching the outstanding *gotipuas* of yesteryears. Gone are the *gurus* and performers of those years.

ROLE OF RAYA RAMANANDA IN *PARAMPARA*

Although Jayadeva's *Gita Govinda* written in 12th century is the first composition on *Radha Krishna Bhava* which has prescribed *raga* and *tala* for each *astapadi*, and, therefore, must have had an impact on dance and music tradition of Orissa, it is generally believed that the person to have a significant influence on the tradition at mass scale was Raya Ramananda Patnaik. Raya Ramananda was the author of the Sanskrit drama *Jagannathballav*.

Raya Ramananda was the minister of King Prataprudra Deva. The kingdom of Prataprudra Deva was spread from Godavari to Ganga and later extended from Triveni in the North to Rameshwar in South. To protect the southern part of his kingdom, Prataprudra Deva had sent Ramananda to Rajamahendri as the Governor. During this time, Shri Chaitanya came to Orissa (1510 AD). Raya Ramananda was a *Vaishnava* and coming in contact with Shri Chaitanya, leaned more and more towards devotional activities. Being with him, Prataprudra Deva also came under the strong influence of Shri Chaitanya so much so that the devotional activities weakened the administrative activities, finally leading to the surrender of Prataprudra to Muslims. However, a cultural revolution occurred under Shri Chaitanya – Ramananda influence. Raya Ramananda was especially skilled in music and dance (Devi, 1963; Das, 1978).

The activities of Raya Ramananda have been documented in the book *Chaitanya Charitamruta* (Goswami, 1984). It is clear from the document that the worship of gods and goddesses through songs, dance and drama was popularised by Raya Ramananda. There is an interesting reference to the fact that he used to teach dance and music to the *devadasis* (obviously belonging to the Jagannath temple). Apparently, he used to compose his own songs and train the *devadasis* for performances. He also taught his own *Jagannathballav Natak* to *devadasis*. A detailed description has been given in *Chaitanya Charitamruta* to the effect that he taught the songs of the drama and also taught them *abhinaya* to these songs. He taught the *Sanchari, Satwika* and *Sthayibhava* to these *devadasis*. It refers to the fact that after they performed before Lord Jagannath, they ate and were sent to their respective homes. Ramananda was an expert in enacting *gopibhava* so much so that the *Vaishnava* poets have referred to him as the *Sakhi Bisakha* of Radha.

Thus, Raya Ramananda was perhaps the first person to bring *maharis* out of the boundary of the temple and trained them the intricacies of *abhinaya*. He also engaged them for playing the feminine roles in the drama *Jagannathballav Natak*.

To conclude, the *parampara* which started as a ritual of the *maharis (devadasis)* in the temple, migrated to the public through *gotipuas*, initially restricted to a specific class but gradually, with the adoption of the art by educated girls from *sambhranta* (aristrocratic) families, developed into one of the best classical dance forms in India.

REFERENCES

Anonymous. *Star of Utkal*, 1912. March 16, pp. 126-27.

Chhamu Chitau (see Appendix 2).

Das, Pandit Nilakantha. 1958. "Hints on the Significance and History of Jagannath", *The Orissa Historical Research Journal*, Vol. VII, April, 1958, Part I, pp. 24-25.

Das, R.K., 1978. "Legends of Jagannath Puri", *Pragati Udyog*, Bhadrak, pp. 95-101.

Devi, Sarala, 1963. *Raya Ramananda* (in Oriya), Orissa Sahitya Academy, Bhubaneswar.

Gargabatu, Pandit Ratnakara, 1933. *Brahmeswar Shilalipi* (in Oriya).
Ghose, M.M. *The Natyasashtra* (undated), *sloka* 60-61, Chapter XXXIV, p. 207.
Goswami, Krushnadas, 1984. *Chaintanya Charitamruta* (edited by H. Mukherjee and S.C. Majumdar), Debasahitya Kutir Pvt. Ltd., Calcutta.
Hunter, W.B., 1872. *Orissa*, Smith, Elder & Co., London.
Khokar, Mohan, 1985. *My Initiation, Souvenir of Angahar Festival*, New Delhi.
Kothari, Sunil, 1965. *Sangeet Natak-8*, Gotipua dancers of Orissa. pp. 32.
Mahapatra, Kedarnath in Souvenir on Late Kedarnath Mahapatra. 1988. Kedarnath Gaveshana Pratisthan, Bhubaneswar.
Mishra, K., 1971. *The Cult of Jagannatha*, Firma K.L. Mukhopadhya, Calcutta.
Mohanty, B., 1958. *Shri Jagannathanka Seba O' Sebaka* (in Oriya), Shri Jagannath Publishers, Bhubaneswar.
O'Malley, L.S.S., 1908. *Bengal District Gazetteers*, Puri, pp. 102-104.
Panigrahi, K.C., 1960. *Kala Vikash Kendra Souvenir*, p. 17.
Pathak, V.S., 1958. "Ekamra-Bhubaneswar in Inscriptions", *The Orissa Historical Research Journal*, VII (1): 47-50.
Pattanaik, D.N., 1974. *Odissi Dance*, Orissa Sangeet Natak Academy, Bhubaneswar.
Praharaj, Gopal Chandra, 1928. *Introduction to Kabisurya Granthabali and Jibanacharita* (in Oriya), Cuttack Printing House, Cuttack.
Purnachandra Oriya Bhashakosha. 1932. Compiled by Gopai Chandra Praharaj, Part 2. Bhashakosha Ashram, Cuttack.
Purnachandra Oriya Bhashakosha, 1934. Compiled by Gopal Chandra Praharaj, Part 4. Bhashakosha Ashram, Cuttack.
Rajguru, Satyanarayana, 1977. "Odissare Nrutya and Sangitara Moulikata" (in Oriya), *Oriya lokanatya*, edited by Rajanikanta Das, Cultural Academy, Rourkela, pp. 1-9.
—, (undated), *Inscriptions of Orissa*.
—, 1978. "Odissara Sangitara Aitihasika-vitti". Seminar on Odissi dance (in Oriya), Orissa Sangeet Natak Academy, pp. 50-55.
Record-of-Rights. 1952. Shri Jagannath Temple, Puri (see Appendix 1).

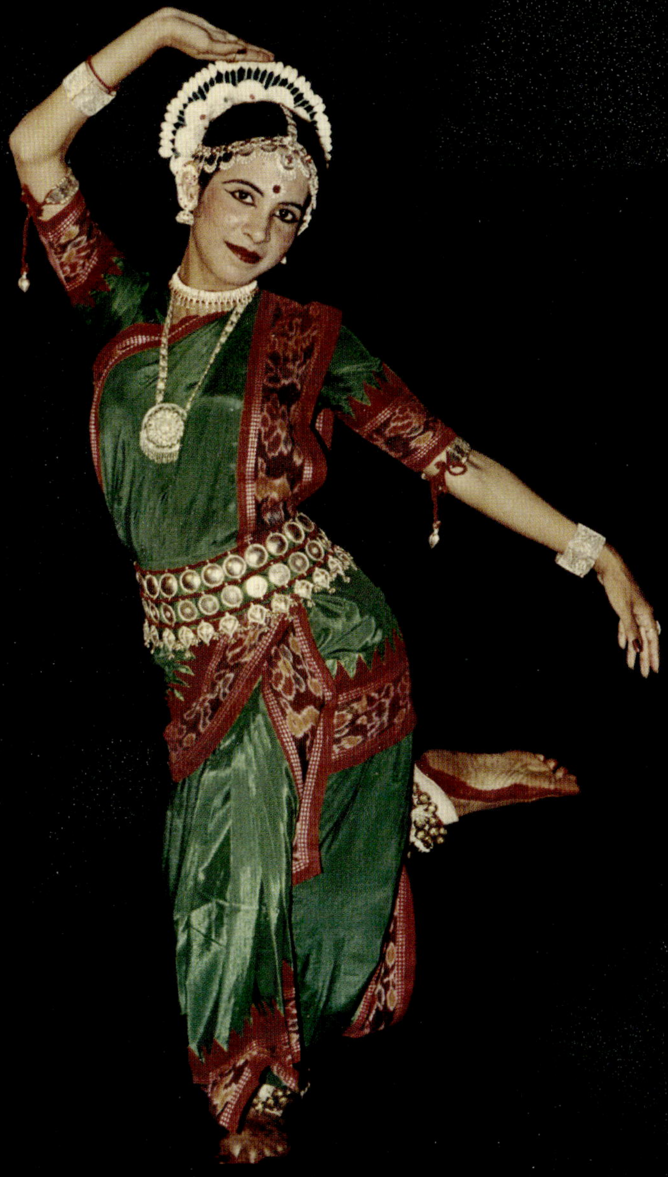

THE REVIVAL 3

Quite, quite sudden and unannounced, it exploded on the world dance scene. Odissi and virtually overnight, emerged a conqueror. This transpired a mere three decades ago, in the early fifties. The high point of the drama is that until then no one outside Orissa had the faintest clue to the existence of the glorious tradition whose praises were now to be sung with a vengeance. And in Orissa itself, though the tradition had blood coursing through its veins, the pulse was feeble, erratic, terminal. If the people accepted the legacy, it was apologetically (Khokar, 1985).

This chapter begins with the introduction of Khokar because it sums up the dramatic revival of Odissi in a relatively short span of time. It also indicates the fact that the dance form was totally unknown outside Orissa. So as a person who got involved (unconsciously initially but consciously at a later stage) in its revival, it is best to document the state of the art as it was in the early part of this century.

As indicated in the part dealing with the *maharis*, nobody really knows when the performances at the Jagannath temple stopped, but during the post-independence period, one could see the *gotipuas* performing fairly regularly during festivals as well as for pure entertainment.

Since the revival is in many ways related to my (Priyambada's) performance in the Youth Festival in New Delhi, in 1954 , I document the background of my training in dance which also gives an insight into the cultural atmosphere of Orissa in the 40's and 50's. However, I must be excused for making this read like an autobiographical account.

Dance was an unknown art form in the traditional Oriya families in the early 1940's. It was something that was exclusively practised by the *gotipuas* who used to tour as professional parties enjoying the patronage of *zamindars*. As mentioned earlier, my paternal grandfather Late Shri Jagabandhu Mohanty, who was a *zamindar* in Jajpur (formerly Cuttack) district and a patron of this art form, maintained a *gotipua* troupe which used to perform in ours as well as nearby villages. In any case, dance and music were generally looked down upon and this is evident from the Oriya proverb *Salaja baé nirlaja gaé, ati alajuka nachaku jaé* which can be loosely translated as "one with modesty plays instrumental music, one with no shame sings and the most shameless of all dances." It is implicit that as in other parts

FACING PAGE :

TOP LEFT :
Priyambada Mohanty dressed in gotipua style, Chauka, 1952.

TOP RIGHT :
Priyambada Mohanty, Bhasa, 1952.

BOTTOM LEFT :
Priyambada Mohanty, Adabhangi.

BOTTOM RIGHT :
Priyambada Mohanty, Chali.

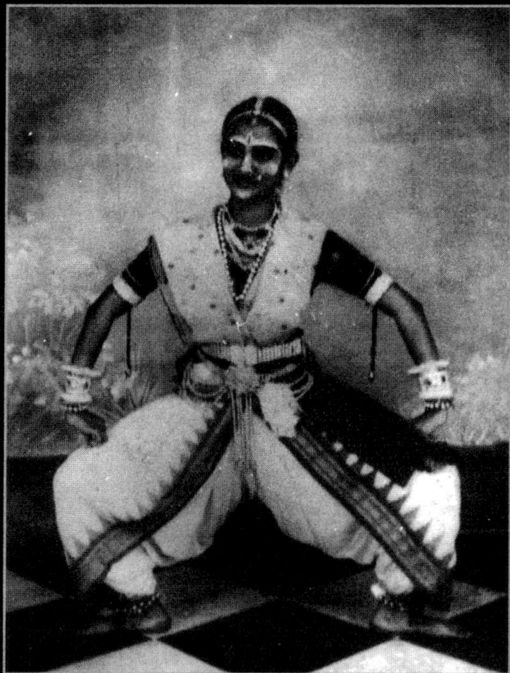
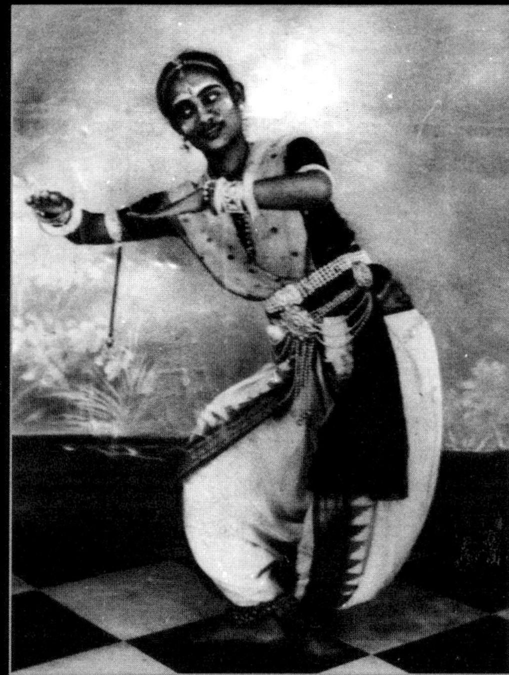
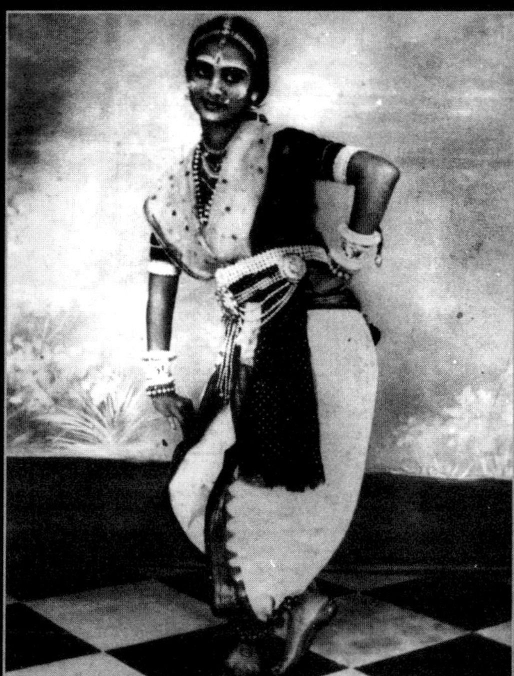
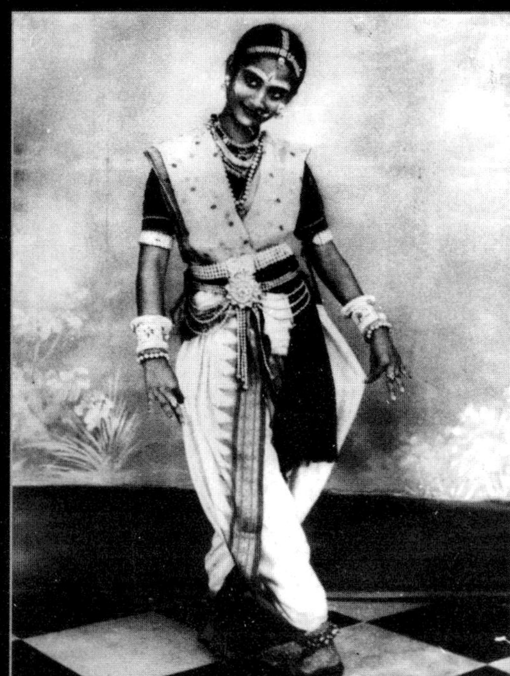

of India, dance was mostly practised by those who were not respected by the contemporary society of the 1940's. Therefore, my learning to dance was more of a freak than the practice of the day. In the early 1940's, a Bengali dance teacher, Shri Banbehari Maity, from Midnapur arrived in Cuttack to make a living as a dance teacher. Little did he know that Oriya girls just did not learn dance. Of course, this was a time when love for music and specially dance in Bengal, had been sparked by people like Uday Shanker and promoted by Gurudev Shri Rabindranath Tagore. Orissa being a neighbouring state, he thought people must be interested in learning dance and therefore he came to Cuttack–the centre for cultural activities in those days. Of course, Utkal Sangeet Samaj had been started as early as 1933 and people were taking interest in teaching children music but nobody danced. My father and some of his contemporaries took pity on him and hired him as a dance teacher more to rehabilitate him than to teach their daughters dancing. This is how dance entered the aristocratic families and Maity gave lessons in about half a dozen of them. He was a good organiser of cultural shows in which we did dance-dramas on the theme of Radha and Krishna. My learning Odissi was even more dramatic. My parents being great patrons of art and literature, took an active interest in the cultural scene in Cuttack. My mother was an executive body member of Utkal Sangeet Samaj where I was a pupil of the *doyen* of Odissi music, Late *Singhari* Shyam Sundar Kar, popularly known as *Singhari*. A few days before the annual function of the school, *Singhari* called me and asked if I was having dance lessons at home. When I replied in the affirmative, much to my surprise he said that he would teach me a special dance for the annual function. I was astounded to say the least as up to then, none of us even dreamt that *Singhari* could dance. The experience of learning Odissi dance from him was unconventional. His dance teaching was unique – he gave lessons from a sitting position. The steps were demonstrated, very clearly, with the hands, and the postures, *mudras*, etc. were acted out waist-up. It was only when he got frustrated with my inability to pick up, would he get up and dance it out for me. This always stunned me because he was so good at it. My ex-teacher, Shrimati Rajarani Ray, who was actively associated with Utkal Sangeet Samaj often said she failed to understand how anyone could translate the mostly verbal instructions of *Singhari* into dance. This has become a matter of pure fun in my family that whatever way I interpreted *Singhari's* instructions "ultimately became the classical Odissi dance". The dance was pure dance without any *abhinaya* and lasted from 5 to 10 minutes. *Singhari* was a master *pakhawaj* player and used to accompany me for my performances. Of course, my first performance was another experience worthy of mention here. *Singhari* insisted that I wear my mother's 14-yard marriage *saree* with a *kachha* in what is known as *dakhsini* (South Indian) style, with the end of the *pallu* pinned to the blouse at the back which lets the *pallu* hang loose. The make-up consisted of a bowl of sandalwood paste into which he dipped his fingers and before I knew what was happening, I had two striped cheeks and a matching forehead. When I objected to my unusual make-up, he cut me short by saying that it was the customary make-up of *maharis*, the dancers in Jagannath temple and therefore, I need not make a fuss about it. I was allowed my mother's golden jewellery for the neck and head, and silver jewellery for the arms. It is an Oriya tradition that we did not wear silver jewellery above the waist as silver was not a metal fit to be worn above the waist in the higher caste. Interestingly enough, I still carry on that tradition because I still use gold jewellery for my neck and head although somewhere along the line gold jewellery was dispensed with for silver jewellery by dancers, probably to harmonize with the silver jewellery on the arms and waist. *Singhari* used to come to stage dressed traditionally in the manner in which he used to do his *seva* (his title *Singhari* came from his duty of dressing Lord Jagannath during the evening, known as *Badasinghara Vesha*). He used to keep the audience spellbound with his regal presence and commanding *pakhawaj* playing. It is a pity that we do not have recordings of his *pakhawaj* for the younger generations to admire. My occasional dances became very popular and soon I was performing in other cultural events also. After one such performance, the late Mr. Asaf Ali, the then Governor of Orissa, gave me an award of Rs. 50/- (then a large sum for a little girl). In any case, *Singhari* was a very important person in the history of development of Odissi music and dance and I feel privileged that I had learnt both the forms of culture from him.

By the late 1940's, more girls had started learning Odissi, and Odissi dance competitions were held at the state level under the auspices of Utkal Sangeet Samaj. By that time other *gurus* had migrated to Cuttack, namely Guru Pankaj Charan Das, Kelucharan Mohapatra and Debaprasad Das who were mainly associated with the Annapurna theatre. Dance was regularly performed in theatres in which Shrimati Laxmipriya, the wife of Guru Kelucharan Mohapatra, was a regular performer. Durllav Chandra Singh, one of the dance teachers in Annapurna theatre at that time told me that he took some of the *bols* (rhythmic syllables) from *Singhari* after seeing my dance and incorporated them in his dance compositions. Due to the efforts of a youth group, an annual festival called the *Kumar Utsab* was started in 1952 at Cuttack. This generated a lot of interest in music and dance. I used to give solo Odissi dance performance in the festival. Then came the 1954 Inter-University Youth Festival, in New Delhi. I had the privilege of being selected to compete in the classical dance category, as Late Shri Shyam Sundar Dhir, the music teacher attached to Ravenshaw College, and Late *Kabichandra* Kalicharan Patnaik thought that I should represent the State. *Singhari* was spending more and more time in Puri and was not associated with dance anymore. At the suggestion of *Kabichandra*, Guru Debaprasad Das accompanied me as my *guru*. *Kabichandra*, the father of modern drama, was also a *vidwan* in dance and music. He took an active interest in my performance and even composed a special song *Gumana Kahinki*, for my *abhinaya*. The perfomance was for about 6-8 minutes, and consisted of a short *sthayi* followed by the *abhinaya* and a short *mokshya*. Going to Talkatora Garden, the venue of the festival, was not a comfortable experience. Stepping out of Orissa for the first time was a little unnerving for me. In addition, in the friendly atmosphere of Talkatora Garden everyone who heard about my style of classical dance asked the same question "What is it"?

Feeling rather insecure after hearing such remarks, I went on stage. Everybody tried their best to make my performance successful. Krishna Babu (Krishna Chandra Ratha), the owner of the biggest enterprise for theatre supplies in Orissa, a singer-dancer-actor in theatre in his young days, did my make-up which lasted for almost two hours. I went on stage dressed in *dakshini* style. The dress consisted of a black velvet blouse with *zari* trimmings

FACING PAGE : *Priyambada Mohanty, dressed in mahari style, 1955.*

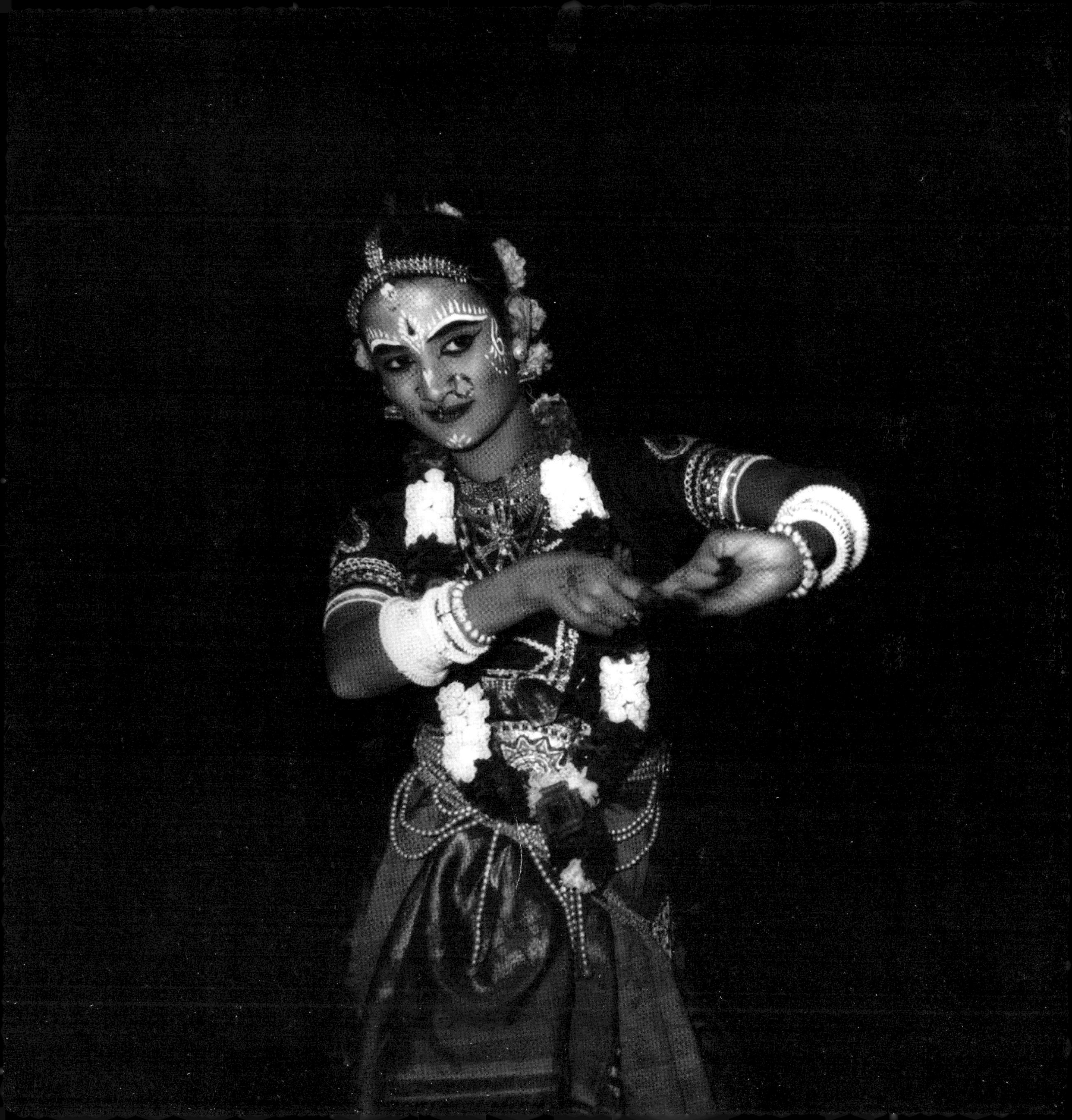

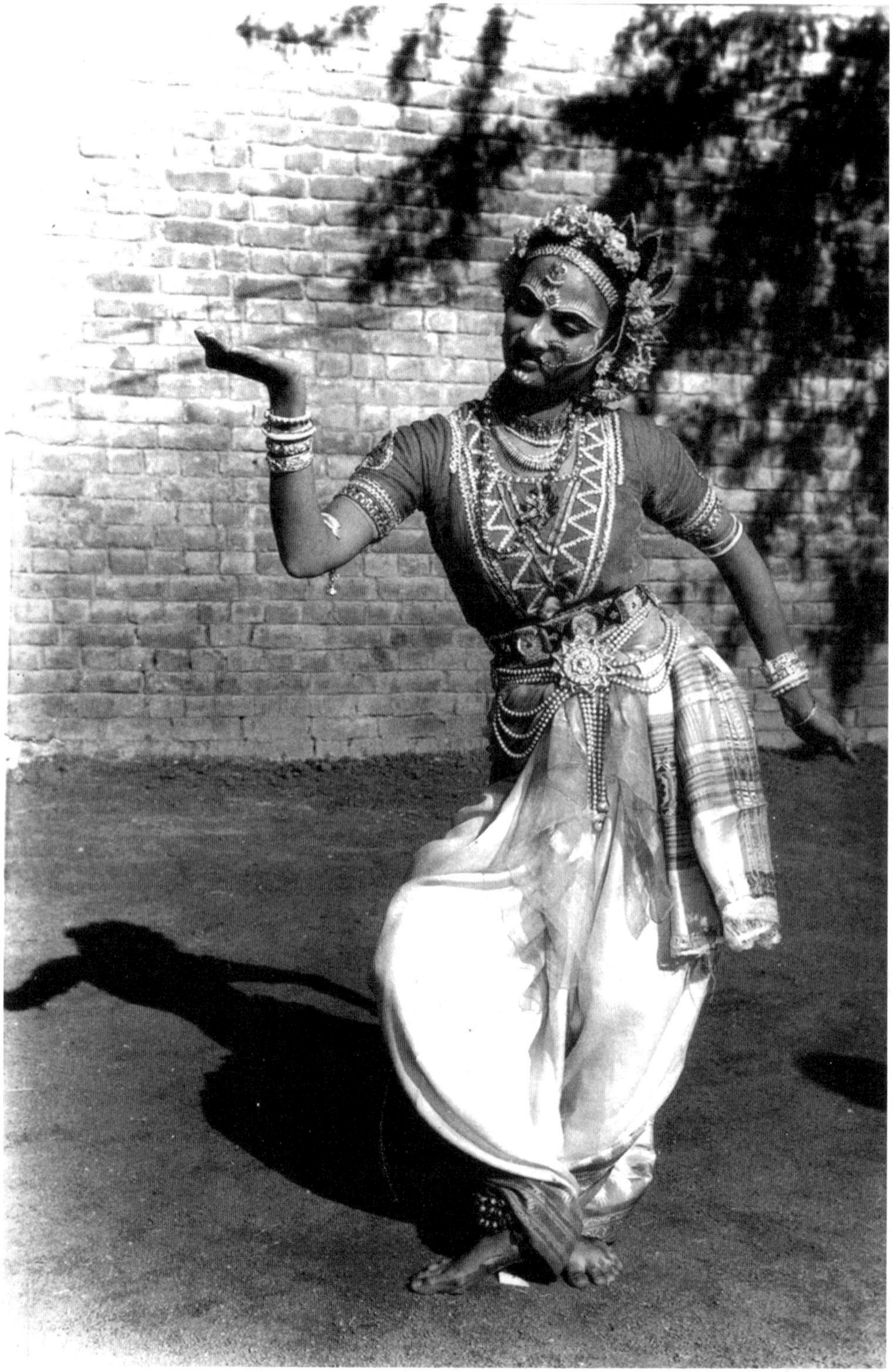

Priyambada Mohanty, dressed in mahari style, 1956 (Inter-University Youth Festival).

and a white *Cuttacki saree* with a black border. Of course, I wore golden jewellery for my neck and head, and silver jewellery on my arms and waist. The reception was stunning. At that moment I did not realise that I was creating history for the revival of Odissi dance. Nobody asked what it was anymore. Our fellow delegates from Bengal admitted that everything from the dance to make-up was *darun* (stunning). I went to the stage as insecure as any dancer in a hostile atmosphere can be, but came out as confident as any "seasoned performer." Many people wanted to know more about it and my fellow delegates and many Oriyas from New Delhi who attended the performance were simply elated.

Most important of all, the performance caught the attention of a lot of important people including the late Dr. Charles Fabri who wrote in the *Statesman* that *there was a strikingly original Odissi dance by Kumari Priyambada Mohanty, obviously a born dancer*. The well-received performance was followed by a lot of speculation whether I should be considered for a prize at all as I had performed in a hitherto unknown style. Bracketed first prizes were given to a *Bharat Natyam* and a *Kathak* dancer, and I was given a third prize; the second prize was not awarded. Although a third prize did not give the best of feelings, it still was a landmark that I bagged a prize at a National level competition by performing an unknown style, paving the way for the recognition of Odissi (Appendix 3). From that day started the long drawn process of official recognition for the dance form. Scholars like *Kabichandra* Kalicharan Patnaik and Shri Dhirendranath Patnaik (who also performed the *dashavatar* in the same youth festival and got a second prize in male category), came out with evidence from the *shastras*. Schlolars, *gurus* and performers came together under the banner "Jayantika" and standardized the sequence and contents of each part. Within one year of my performance, we were invited to perform in the Dance Festival at New Delhi. Under the dynamic leadership of the executive committee members and the vice president, Late Shrimati Nisamoni Devi (my mother), of the newly constructed Utkal Nrutya Sangeeta Natyakala Parishad (now renamed as the Sangeet Natak Akademi), Guru Pankaj Charan Das and Guru Kelucharan Mohapatra choreographed the dance drama *Sakhigopal* by *Kabichandra. Kabichandra* composed a *Mangalacharan* "*Padabande Gananatha*" for me which has become

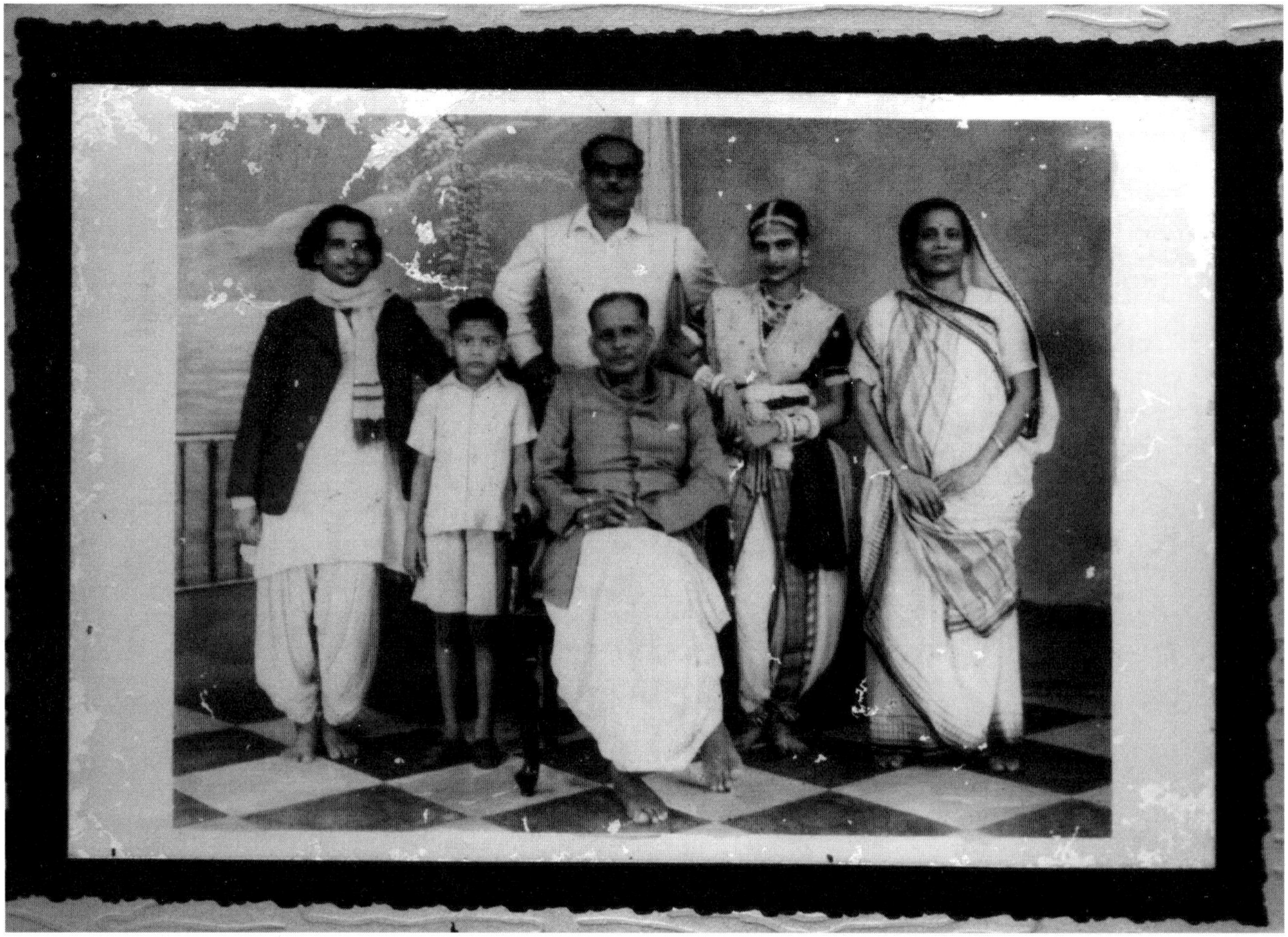

Group with Guru Debaprasad Das (standing left), Kabichandra Kalicharan Patnaik (sitting), Priyambada Mohanty standing next to her mother Shrimati Nisamoni Devi on the right.

a traditional piece for Odissi now. By 1956, in the third Inter-University Youth Festival, Odissi had been classified as a separate dance form. I won the first prize representing Lucknow University. Odissi being unknown then, the style has been mentioned as "Oriya" in one of my certificate (Appendix 4). In the meantime, Shrimati Indrani Rehman came to Orissa in 1957 and wanted to learn Odissi. Guru Debaprasad Das became her teacher and Indrani carried Odissi outside India. She has described her role in Odissi revival and her association with Guru Shri Debaprasad Das in detail (Rahman, 1993). In addition, she has also documented how the interest of her husband

(Habib Rahman) who saw me dance in Delhi, and the encouragement of Dr. Charles Fabri were critical for her learning Odissi dance.

However, it still remained for Odissi to make a mark as a self- sufficient dance form. Under the patronage and persevering interest of Dr. Fabri and the late Dr. Mayadhar Mansinha, I finally gave a full evening performance at Sapru House in Delhi, on October 14 and 15, 1961 (Appendix 5), under the auspices of the Little theatre Group headed by Shri Inder Lall Dass. The programme consisted of *abhinaya* to traditional Oriya songs including one each from Kabisurya, Banamali and Gopalakrishna, three pieces from the *Gita Govinda* and two *pallavis*, *batu*, *mangalacharan*, and *mokshya.* Late Pandit Banambara Acharya translated *Gita Govinda* into Oriya and Dr. Mansinha translated all the songs into English which were printed in the programme. Kelu Sir (Guru Kelucharan Mohapatra) choreographed the dances, and Balakrishna Das set the music for some pieces. In addition to Guru Kelucharan Mohapatra and Balakrishna Das, flutist Shri Raghunath Seth and violinist Shri Arun Kumar Chaudhury provided the accompaniment. The programme was well received and Odissi finally proved to be a self-sustaining dance form.

I was rather surprised to find Mrs. Indira Gandhi present among the audience. At the end of the performance, Dr. Fabri told me that Mrs. Gandhi had come at his request to encourage me and the cause of Odissi which was struggling to make its mark, but she had to leave with a request to convey her regrets for not staying till the end of the perfomance because her son had a temperature. I then got a glimpse into the many levels of her personality. She came to encourage an unknown dancer (me) performing an almost unknown struggling dance form (Odissi) in spite of the fact that her son was not well. It also gave me an insight into what a loving and caring mother she was, to have come for only a short time, returning early to be with him. A few days later, I was even more pleasantly surprised to receive a personal letter from her, telling me how much she enjoyed my dancing and wishing me and Odissi dance success in the future. Madam Gandhi had the *Midas* touch–Odissi flourished and rose to be recognised as a very popular classical dance form.

Soon after I repeated part of the programme for the delegates of the

Indian Science Congress held at Cuttack in 1962, *Prajatantra*, a leading newspaper of Cuttack commented that:

> Priyambada Mohanty kept the audience spellbound with her Odissi recital; it has not been possible for anybody so far to perform Odissi for such a long time in one stretch.

The accompanists for this programme were the best one could ever get; in addition to Kelu Sir and Balakrishna Das, Hariprasad Chaurasia played the flute and Shri Bhubaneswar Mishra the violin. With the excellent reviews, invitations to perform in other parts of India followed. However, Odissi *gurus* were reluctant to travel then. It meant performing with substitute accompanists or playing the tape in the background. I tried both and both were disappointing. In my first performance at the Rashtrapati Bhavan in 1956, I was doing *mokshya* barely 5 feet away from Pandit Jawaharlal Nehru and Brezhnev, when suddenly the sound of *pakhawaj* stopped. Then to my horror, I discovered the *pakhawaj* rolling towards me. With a quick side step, I picked it up, chanted the *ukutas* and with a typical Odissi *chali*, handed over the *pakhawaj* to Shri Banabehari Moharana. Fortunately, he took the cue and played from where he had left off without a hitch. Shri Moharana is the cousin of Kelu Sir and since he could not go, he sent his cousin brother with me. Now, of course, things have changed; Banabehari Moharana is one of the most sought-after *pakhawaj* players and often jokingly refers to his first accompaniment with me, and how I recovered the *pakhawaj* from under the noses of two chiefs of countries. Playing with tapes was also discouraging.

It would be unfair if I do not mention the incomparable contribution of Dr. Charles Fabri to Odissi dance. He not only gave wide publicity to the dance form but also gave us the self confidence to tide over all the obstacles and criticisms that were levelled against Odissi as a self-sufficient dance form. I feel it is appropriate that I give Fabri's introduction to my full evening performance to capture the spirit of Fabri in the struggle for recognition of Odissi.

There are still some naive people who go on believing that there are four classical systems of dancing in India– Bharata Natya, Kathakali, Kathak and Manipuri. This is an entirely incorrect and untenable belief, and I have effectively exploded this myth in an article I wrote for the special number devoted to Orissi dance by *Marg* magazine. A much more likely figure is eight; but it is not impossible that a few more classical systems will be discovered in this vast land in which a system as superb, as admirable, as classic in its rules and as rich in its powers of expressions as Orissi is, had to wait until in 1954 I had the good luck to announce its "discovery". It has been known to be sure to Oriyas but not outside Orissa.

In fact, the great textbook writer, Bharata, whose Natya-sastra is the most thorough treatise on the arts of dance, theatre and music, mentions that in his days (probably the 2nd or 1st century BC), there existed a system of dance in Orissa and Bihar ("Odhra-Magadhi" as he calls it), and all of us ought to have observed much earlier that some such system of dancing must have existed in Orissa at least from around 600 AD, as all of us knew that the hundreds of temples of Orissa are replete with relievo carvings showing dancers in all sorts of poses and that from the earliest temples at Bhubaneswar (Baital Deul, Parasurameswar, c. 600-650 AD) to the Sun temple of Konarka (dedicated in 1250 AD).

The fact, however, is that Orissi, contrary to Bharata Natya, was never danced anywhere but in one single place; in front of Lord Jagannatha, in the great temple of Puri; although here and there the "gotipuas" (young boy acrobat dancers) did learn a good deal of Orissi as part of their trade.

A quick definition of classical dance is that it is handed down from teacher to pupil and has strict rules; whereas folk dance is learnt by any dancer who likes to join the frolic, without a teacher and with no set rules. Orissi possesses all the four elements of classical dance set down by Bharata (Manipuri does not posses these elements) and is a close relation of the Bharata Natya and Kuchipudi systems of dancing. There are reasons to postulate based on inner evidence that Orissi is a purer and older edition of Bharata Natya, less codified, less punditic and that it preserves a tradition certainly identical with that depicted on the ancient temple walls of Orissa.

The extant Oriya textbooks go back at least to the 14th century and as palm leaf manuscripts do not last very long, this is a respectable antiquity enough. There is nevertheless, no possible doubt that these manuscripts are based on

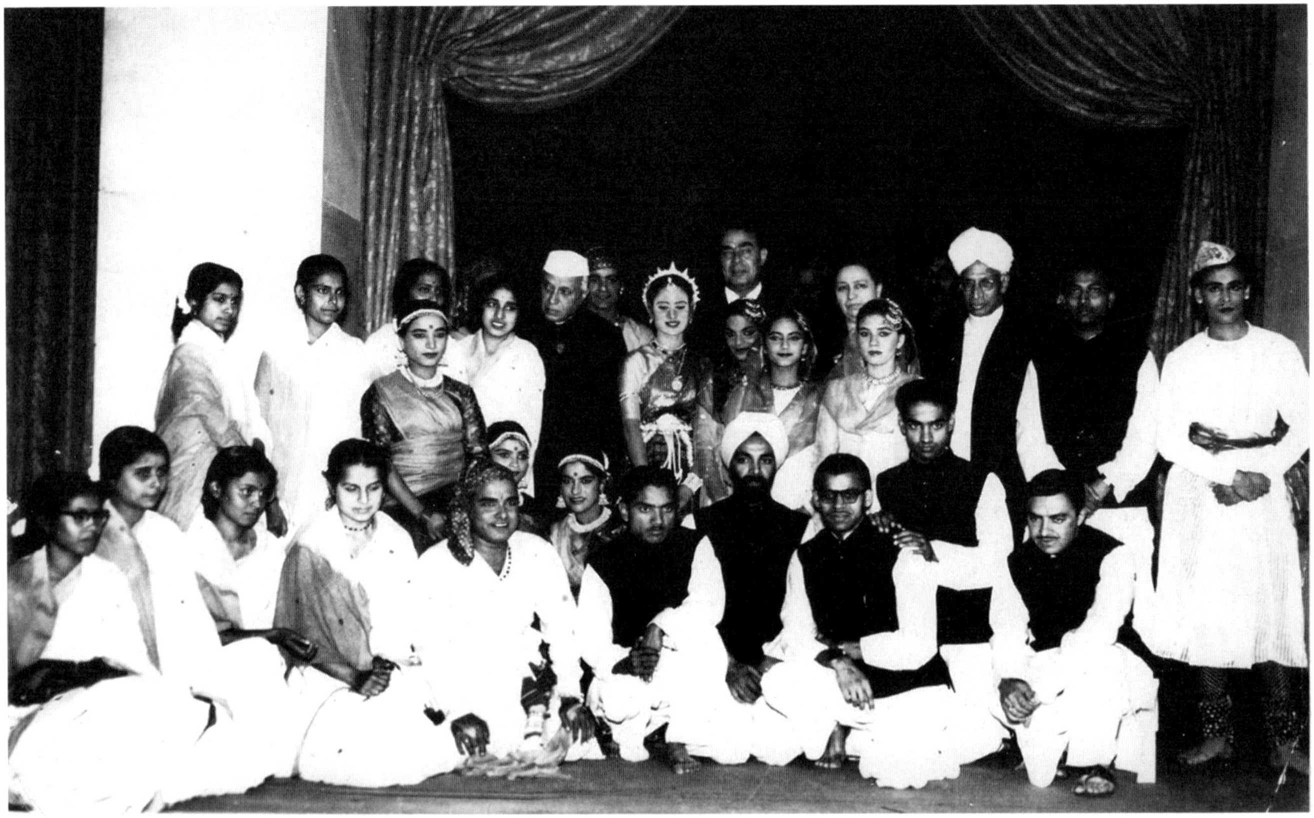

Rashtrapati Bhavan Programme, Priyambada in between Pandit Nehru and Breznev, 5.12.1961.

much older texts that have been destroyed with the passage of time. The climate of Orissa is not conducive to longevity in dried palm leaves.

Now that Orissi has come out of the Jagannatha temple, a number of schools are teaching Orissi to girls and boys of good education. Formerly, only the professional classes had knowledge of it and like temple dancing girls elsewhere, their meagre pittance at the temple was not sufficient to support them and society drove them to become kept women. The situation has now greatly changed and Orissi is highly respected and admired by the educated classes of the State.

Ms. Priyambada Mohanty is one of the greatest pioneers, for she went to Puri (there were no teachers at that time in Cuttack) at the age of five to learn Orissi. It was her appearance at the Inter-University Youth Festival in 1954 that first brought Orissi to Delhi. It was shortly after that, that Mrs. Indrani Rehman on

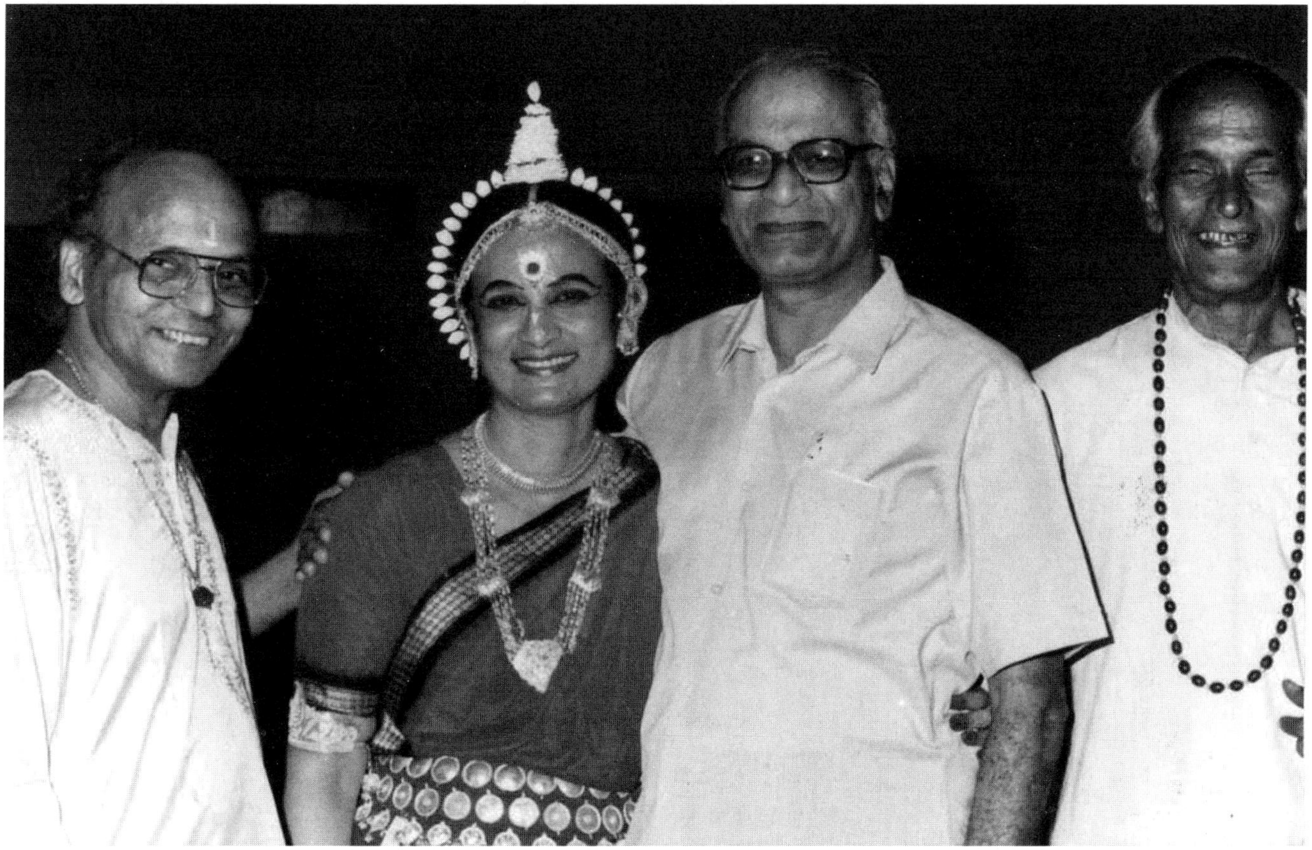

Priyambada with Guru Kelucharan Mahapatra left, Vice-President Central Sangeet Natak Akademi Shri P.V. Krishnamoorthy and Guru Pankaj Charan Das (right), 1987 (courtesy: Central Sangeet Natak Adademi, New Delhi).

my suggestion went to Cuttack to learn Orissi and carried the system triumphantly round half the globe. She is still continuing to dance in the United States.

It has taken a long number of years to convince the old fashioned people of the very existence of this precious heritage of Indian art. One of the most potent reasons is that the young ladies of Orissa who have learnt the art of Orissi dance are not ready to take it up professionally. This, in fact, is the first time that an audience will have the chance to see an Oriya lady in a full evening's programme of Orissi in the capital and observe the wealth and beauty of one of the world's most wonderful styles of classical dancing.

(Fabri, October, 1961)

Fabri also in his own inimitable style initiated a campaign to simplify our elaborate make-up and heavy jewellery (much of which kept falling off

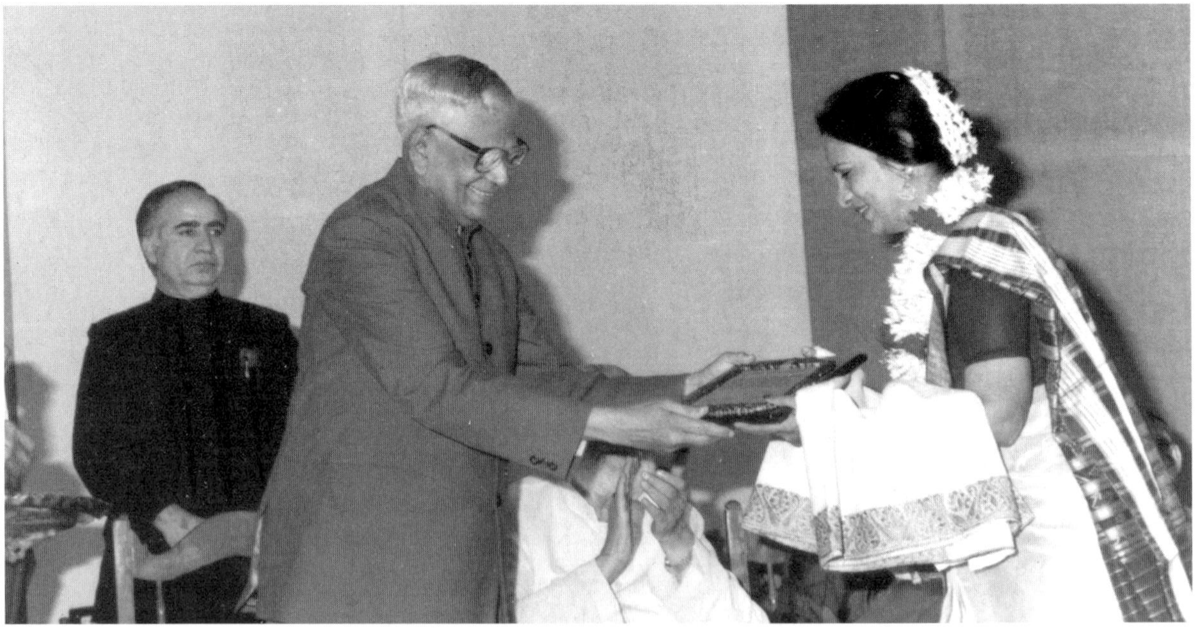

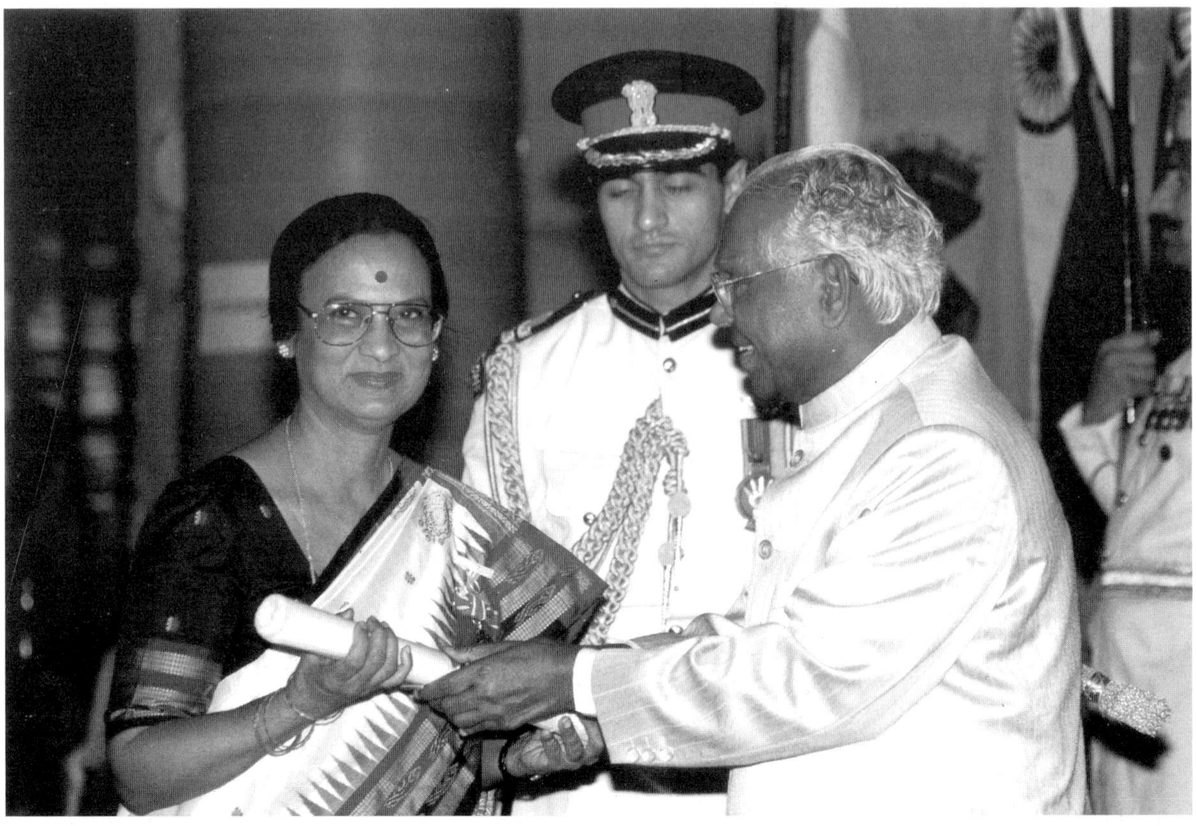

during the performance). He was most critical of our tendency for over-dressing and the ornate make-up with white dots. Needless to say, with Fabri's insistence the dress became more and more elegant and the decoration with white dots finally receded to a few lines around the *bindi.* It appears that despite Fabri's opinion, a few white dots not only stayed with Odissi make-up but they finally became part of the make-up of many leading Kathak, Bharat Natyam and Kuchipudi dancers. Another contribution of Odissi to make-up is that of the Kali (few strands of hair styled on the side of cheeks, in front of the ear). I remember Habib Saheb (Indrani's husband) saying that it looked very nice and he could not tell through his opera glasses whether it was real hair or make-up. Even the dress underwent many changes. Initially, I used to wear the *saree* in *Dakshini* style. In 1955, I discovered the graceful *mahari* style which I adopted for many of my performances. The *mahari* style is unique to Odissi only. It consists of a *kanchala* (blouse with trimmings which is tied at the back) and a *saree* wrapped in a distinctive style from the waist down called *Kania kachha.* From the *gotipuas* came the style which resembles that of Bharat Natyam and we had a choice of tucking the decorative *anchal* at the side or in the front like a fan.

The jewellery have been simplified to a few pieces of which the most distinctive is the *Benga-patia* waist band. Another distinctive jewellery is the *Ketaki Panapatra Gua*, which means the *ketaki* flower, betel leaf and areca nut (all ingredients of *pan*). This piece of jewellery was meant for decorating the head. However, it is not much in use now.

Odissi repertoire has undergone considerable transformation since the 1940's. Odissi was mainly a continuous dance where the dancer used to stand with folded hands when a *Ganesh struti* was recited. The dance started with what can best be described as the *batu* or *sthayi* then continued into *tarijham (pallavi)* and then into *abhinaya. Abhinaya* was interspersed with pure dance pieces and finally ended in a short *mokshya.* The duration was between 15-20 minutes. My dance at the Ist Inter-University Youth Festival was for 8 minutes and that at the 3rd Inter-University Youth Festival for 14 minutes. But at *Jayantika*, the continuous piece was broken up into different divisions, namely, *mangalacharan*, *batu* (or *sthayi*), *pallavi*, *abhinaya* and *mokshya.* With this separation came the enacting of the *sloka* in praise of

FACING PAGE :

TOP :
Priyambada receiving Central Sangeet Natak Akademi Award from President Honourable Venkataraman (courtesy: Central Sangeet Natak Akademi, New Delhi).

BOTTOM :
Priyambada receiving Padmashri from President K.R. Narayanan

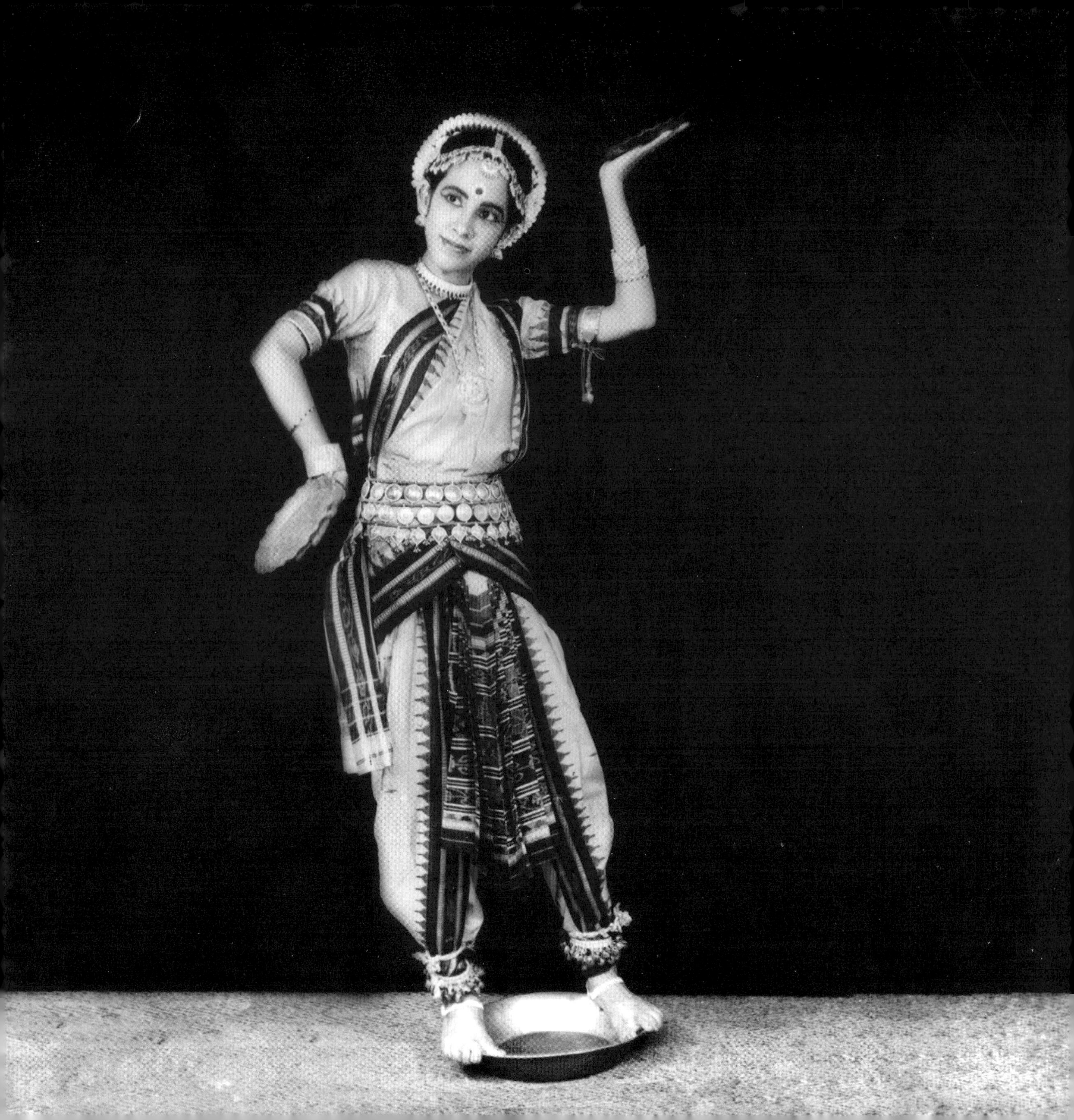

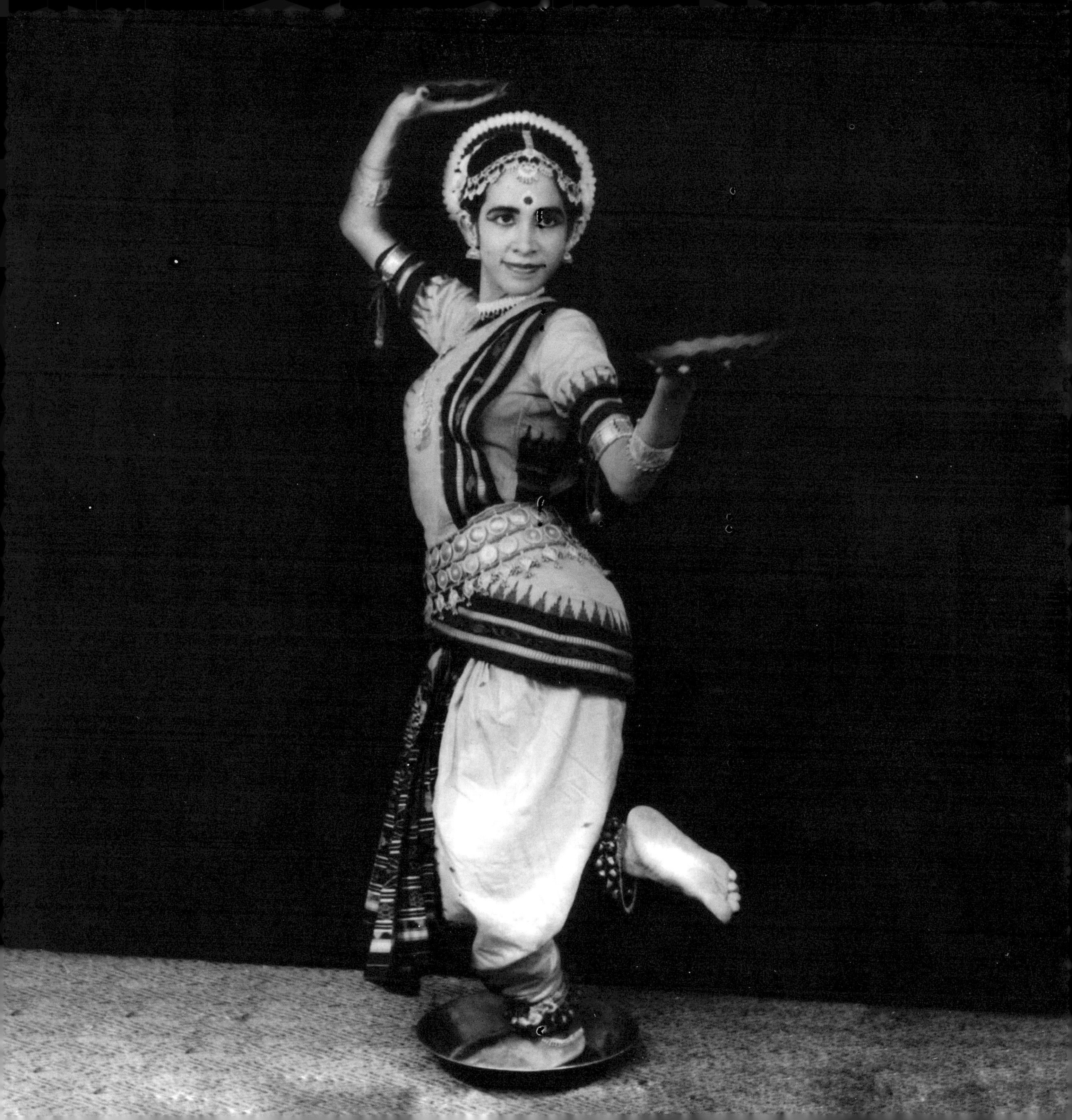

gods and goddesses. Initially, it was restricted to Lord Ganesha. Then Guru Pankaj Charan Das introduced Sankaracharya's *Jagannathastaka-Kadachit Kalindi* which is quite popular now. Interestingly enough, this is often followed with *Ganesha vandana* which is not the proper tradition, as Ganesha is the first one to be worshipped according to Hindu tradition. At present, invocation to *Devi,* Shiva and Vishnu is also done. But, the traditional piece of pure dance (*nritta)* is still maintained ending with a tripartite salutation to the mother earth (for treading on her), to the audience and the musicians.

Batunrutya, which is the most stylized form, is also the most sculpturesque. Here the dancer goes from one sculpturesque pose to another without any rest to the chanting of rhythmic *ukutas*. Interestingly enough, the three leading *gurus* – Guru Pankaj Charan Das, Guru Kelucharan Mohapatra and Guru Debaprasad Das – have three different pieces under the same category with different names (*sthayi*, *batu* and *thai nrutya*, respectively). These three pieces, although basically the same, also show the marks of distinction between the three.

Pallavi, previously known as *tarijham*, has undergone the maximum evolution amongst all the divisions. An item of pure dance, this piece has the maximum scope for variation in music as well as *tala*. Initially, an intricate part leading to *abhinaya* therefore, always in the same *raga* as the *abhinaya (sabhinaya pallavi)*, at present it is mostly performed in a *raga* different from the following *abhinaya*. It is the most graceful item where the dancer interprets the musical patterns beginning from simplistic to complex ones. Initially, it was a 2-3 minute piece and now it has been developed into 10-15 minute items. The emphasis is on *lasya*, and *tribhangas* are used profusely in this item.

Abhinaya is the interpretation of the lyrics by facial expressions and hand gestures. *Abhinaya* was the forte of the *gotipuas* and, therefore, most of the Oriya songs composed by Kabisurya, Gopalakrushna and Banamali were used initially in Odissi. Incorporation of *Gita Govinda* started with the popularisation of the songs through the play *Jayadeva* by Late *Kabichandra* Kalicharan Patnaik. But *Gita Govinda* was used for Odissi only in the late 50's. Of course, the Odissi medium has been so suitable and Guru Kelucharan Mohapatra's choreography so apt, that many believe Odissi to be synonymous

PROCEEDING PAGES :

PAGE 68 :
Ahalya Hejmadi, Thali Nrutya.

PAGE 69 :
Ahalya Hejmadi, Thali Nrutya.

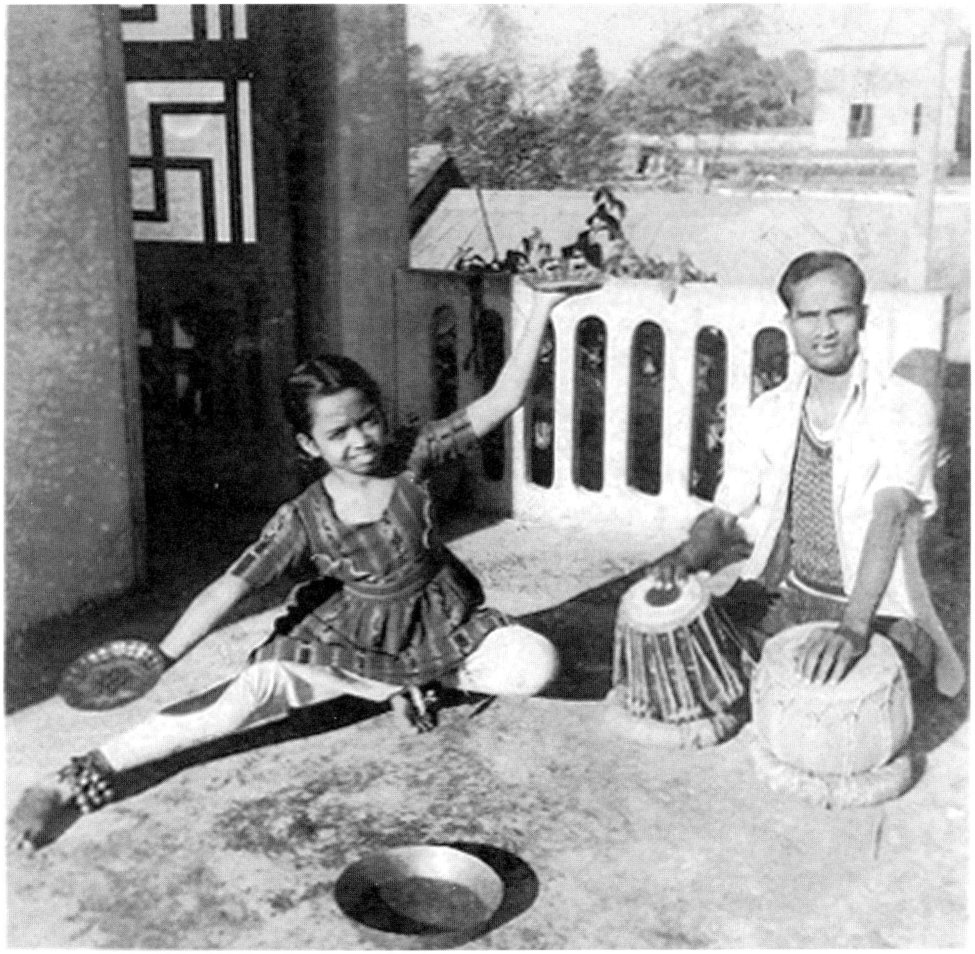

Guru Pankaj Charan Das teaching Thali Nrutya to Madhuri Mohanty, early 1950's.

with *Gita Govinda*. With non-Oriya girls taking up Odissi, *Gita Govinda* was used more frequently than the Oriya songs. But, the depth of Odissi is hardly explored by *Gita Govinda*. Each Oriya song has many levels of interpretations which is not possible with *Gita Govinda*. Therefore, at present there is a reversal to Oriya lyrics which is a good sign. In any case, the lyrical demure of Odissi is a very suitable medium for *abhinaya*. But still there are two distinct styles of *abhinaya* – the *gotipua* and the non-*gotipua* style, out of which the former is more perky and interspersed with spurts of pure dance.

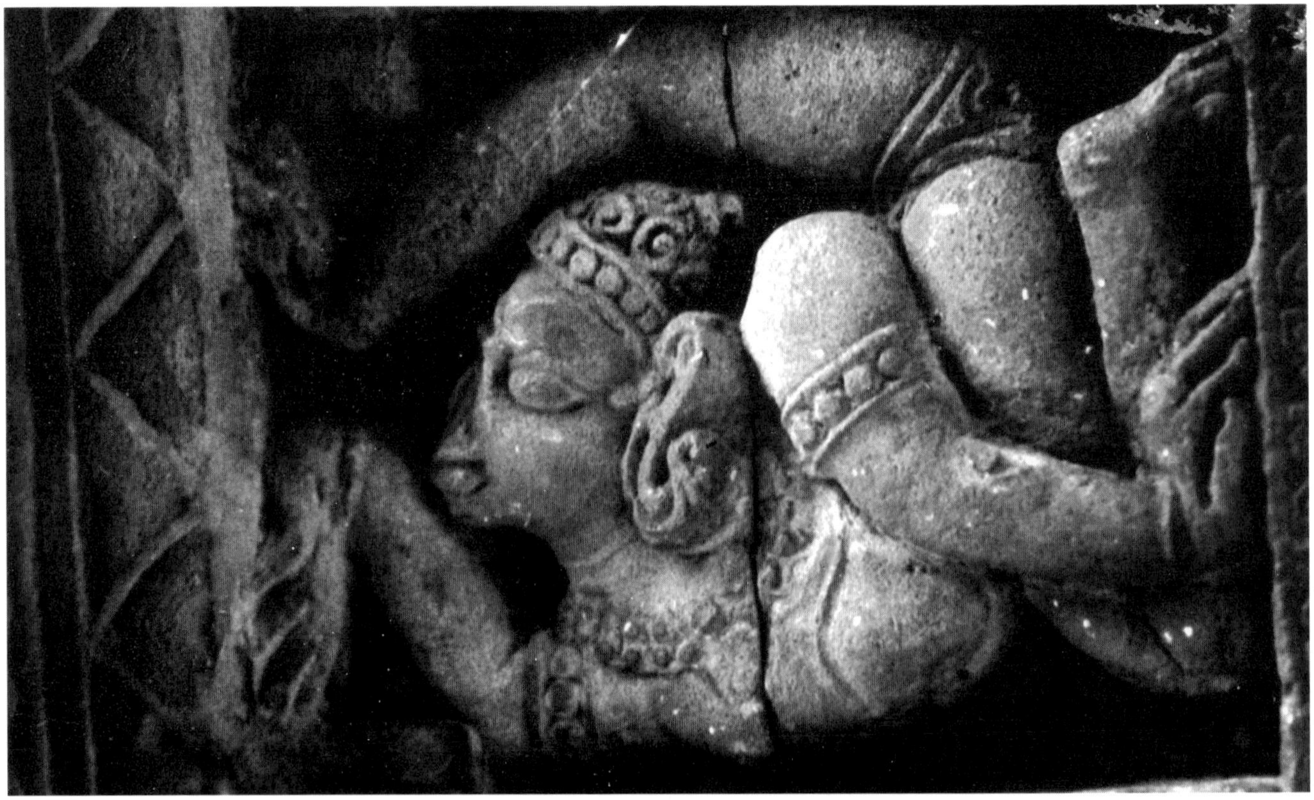

Bandha sculpture from Parasurameswar.

Mokshya is the most interesting item from *tala* point of view. Typical variations of Odissi – *tala-pahapata* and *sariman* – are used in an intricate varying tempo. This item, like *batu*, is very difficult and therefore, not performed as frequently as it should be. It can best be described as the dance of liberation. During recent times, *mokshya* has been topped with narrative *slokas* to highlight the spirit of *mokshya*.

In addition, skilled items like the *Thali Nrutya* and acrobatic items like the *Bandha nrutya* derived from *gotipua* tradition are included in the repertoire.

SONG AND DANCE TRADITION IN ORISSA

The first musically oriented poems in Orissa were the *Bauddha Gana O' Doha*, composed during the 9th to 10th century. Several of these poems were written by Kanhupa, Luipa, Shabaripa, etc. from Orissa and most of the *ragas* mentioned for the poems, namely, *Pattamanjari, Debakri, Ramakeri, Dhanashri*, and *Desakshya* are now used in Odissi music. Thus, these songs represent the earliest tradition of music in Orissa (Das, 1986).

But the tradition of songs as we know it today, perhaps began in the 12th century with the composition of *Gita Govinda* by the immortal poet Jayadeva. The Sanskrit *astapadis* of Jayadeva are unique compositions in the sense that Jayadeva specified *tala* and *raga* for each *astapadi.* In addition, he also has given the *raga lakshanas* in the beginning of some compositions. These Sanskrit songs of *Gita Govinda* are in direct ancestral line of songs and musical poetry in Oriya. The same *ragas* and *talas* are used now although interestingly enough, most of the present-day *astapadi* tunes have changed in time and do not conform to the specific *talas* and *ragas* prescribed by Jayadeva.

It is believed that Jayadeva was born in Kendubilwa in Puri district (Mohapatra, 1973). In the last part of *Gita Govinda,* Jayadeva has mentioned that the name of his father was Bhojadeva and his mother was Rama Devi. He has also mentioned that his wife, Padmavati, was an expert in music and dance. As mentioned in the context of *maharis,* Padmavati is believed to have also been a *devadasi* performing in the temple of Lord Jagannath.

Jayadeva has not mentioned the name of any Raja in his compositions. But it is said that Ekajata Kamadeva or Kamarnaba (1147 to 1157 AD) did not even touch water (meaning food) without listening to the *Gita Govinda.* Based on this, it is believed that Jayadeva must have been a contemporary of Kamarnaba and must have written it before 1157 AD, in the 12th century.

One interesting point that must be made here is that although the *pundits* had given much importance to *Gita Govinda* as an outstanding composition, they were reluctant to introduce it into the rituals of Jagannath temple. Even Kamarnaba who was so fond of *Gita Govinda*, could not introduce it into the rites of the Jagannath temple. But there was no objection to anyone singing it in an informal level in the temple premises.

But gradually, with the popularity of *Gita Govinda* all over Orissa, it could be incorporated into rituals. Ganga ruler Narasinghadeva II (1278-1307 AD) introduced Shri *Gita Gobinda gana seva* in the Jagannath temple (Mahapatra, 1973). In the following period, various factors led to the replacement of *Gita Govinda* by the composition *Abhinaba Gitagobinda* by Shri Purosottama Deva of Solar dynasty (Surya Vansi), famous for conquering Kanchi. This is believed to be part of the politics of languages, Oriya versus Sanskrit, as scholars from each tried to prevail upon the ruler to have rituals conducted in that particular language. But after the death of Purosottama Deva, the Sanskrit *pundits* prevailed upon King Prataprudra Deva, son of Purosottama Deva, to decree that Shri *Gita Govinda* written by Jayadeva only should be recited in *Shree Mandira.* This has been carved on the *Jaya Vijaya dwara* in the Jagannath temple. This was done on 8 July in 1500 AD, on *Bahuda* day (return car festival). Since people from all over India flock to Puri for the car festival, it is believed that the decree spread far and wide and is responsible for the spreading and popularity of Jayadeva's *Gita Govinda* all over India. Even the two deities, *Balabhadra* and *Jagannatha* came to be known as "Shri *Gita Govinda stuta* or *bandita debatas*" (deities). According to the decree from the Gajapati Maharaja to Parikshya (*Parichha*):

a) During each *bhoga* (offering of food) and end of *sandhya dhupa* to *badashringara* (decoration ceremony at night), dance will be performed to the singing of Shri *Gita Govinda* only.

b) *Balabhadra thakura's sampradaya, Kapileswara thakura* associated dancers, old *sampradaya* and *Telenga sampradaya* should learn only Shri *Gita Govinda* and no other songs. During the dance in the presence of *Mahaprabhu*, only Shri *Gita Govinda* will be sung and no other.

c) Apart from these four *sampradayas*, the *Baishnaba* singers should only sing Shri *Gita Govinda.* They will teach only Shri *Gita Govinda* to *ashikhita* (literally meaning illiterate – perhaps novices will be more appropriate).

The *mandira Parichha* who disobeys the Raja's decree and gives permission to sing, as an accompaniment to dance, any other song except Shri *Gita Govinda*, will be a *drohi* (traitor) of *Jagannath.*

Thus, the tradition of regular *Gita Govinda seva* is more than 450 years old. Perhaps this was one way of standardising the music and dance ritual in the temple. Because it is obvious that at least the *Telenga sampradaya* must have found it difficult to recite Oriya lyrics. In any case, the *Gita Govinda seva* later gave way to a means to be indoctrinated as *Gita Govinda sebayat* as mentioned earlier. The present-day *maharis* sing mainly Oriya songs for the ritual and very few songs from *Gita Govinda* (see chapter on Parampara).

In the early 1940's when I started dancing, *gotipuas* danced to the Oriya lyrics of Odissi and Champu. It is perhaps due to the efforts Late *Kabichandra* Kalicharan Patnaik made in staging the successful musical drama *Jayadeva* that *Gita Govinda* became popular in the 40's and 50's. When I prepared for the first full evening's programme in New Delhi, in 1961, I had chosen to dance three pieces from the *Gita Govinda.* Now Odissi has become almost synonymous with *Gita Govinda*. The translations of some of the pieces that were incorporated into Odissi repertoire in the early 60's are given at the end of this chapter. These were translated exclusively for me by Late Dr. Mayadhar Mansinha.

Of the many Oriya composers of Radha-Krishna songs, the three who dominated the field of music and dance, popularly referred to as *the trinity*, are *Kabisurya* Baladeva Rath, Gopalkrushna Patnaik and Banamali Das (née Patnaik). Of these three, *Kabisurya* is the most musical, Gopalkrushna the most poetic, and Banamali the most devotional. Since they still dominate the song-music field in Orissa, it is appropriate to deal with their life and some of their compositions which were translated for me by Late Dr. Mayadhar Mansinha.

Kabisurya Baladeva Rath (1780-1845 AD)

Kabisurya Baladeva Rath, more commonly known as *Kabisurya*, was a poet-administrator (Das, 1987; Patnaik, undated). He was born in 1780 at Vijayanagargarha, the capital of Khemundi State, now in Ganjam district in southern Orissa. Vijaynagargarha was around 10 km from the present-day Digapahandi. Vijayanagargarha was a prosperous town ruled by the most powerful king of the State, Sri Purosottam Anangabhimadeva (1728-1776) of Ganga dynasty. Kabisurya's father was Ujjal Ratha, a *pundit* in his kingdom. Political instability and domestic disputes ultimately led to the division of the town into two parts – Vijayanagargarha (Bada Khemundi) and Pratapgirigarha (Sana Khemundi) – and also disrupted the glory of the royal court. Ujjal Ratha had to earn his living by teaching. Baladeva was born during the hard days of his father. He lost his mother in his childhood and was sent to his maternal grand-father Tripurari Otta, in Athagarha, in Ganjam district. Tripurari Otta was an eminent *pundit* and tantric of his time. He looked after Baladeva well and educated him. After completing his studies, Baladeva returned to his father and got married. He lost his father soon after and fell upon hard times. Fortunately for him the king of the neighbouring State, Sri Rama Chandra Chottray, invited him to boost his image as a patron of art and culture. Baladeva's poetic talent got an opportunity to grow and blossom. The king bestowed upon him the title of *Kabisurya*, which literally means, *the sun among the poets*. Besides being a poet, Baladeva was an accomplished musician and composed his own songs. Catering to the tastes of feudal chiefs, the songs of Baladeva are ornate, flamboyant, colourful and sensuous.

Fortunately for him and ultimately for Oriya literature, his immense creative abilities were readily recognised and applauded. In course of time, he became an able administrator and was appointed as the *Diwan* or chief administrator of the State. As a successful poet-administrator later in his life, he was not only honoured as a great poet by many kings but also enjoyed the priviledge to work as the *Diwan* in several princely States. Even the East India Company appointed him as the manager and royal guardian of Mahuri and Paralakhemundi states, respectively. Kings donated land to him in appreciation of his creative abilities. Free from financial and other mundane worries, his creativity soared and his fame spread all over Orissa. He is one of the lucky ones amongst the Oriya poets as he got both prosperity and laurels during his lifetime. In 1810, at the invitation of the young prince of Athagarha, Baladeva moved to Athagarha. He was appointed both the court poet and *Diwan.* His period of stay there saw the crowning achievement of his poetic genius. Here he composed his famous *Chaupadi Chautisa* and *Kishore Chandrananda Champu*. He also wrote a prose, *Hasya Kallol.* The benevolent king offered him the coveted *Raiguru* title which was usually offered to those who excelled in all *shastras*. This brought him to the notice of Sri Mukunda Deva, the king of Puri who sent the royal certificate of merit to Baladeva. Later on, Mukunda Deva honoured Baladeva in his own court at Puri, as "*Kabisurya Raiguru* Mohapatra". It is believed that

Kabisurya lived at Athagarha from 1810 to 1820. Then as an administrator under the East India Company, he acted as the manager of Mahuri state, in Ganjam district, from 1821 to 1830. He was allotted an important post in Paralakhemundi but left in 1834 to settle down at Berhampur. He built his house at Balajipentha and lived a full life. It is said that in 1845, he went to Athagarha at the invitation of his friend, the King of Athagarha, where he contracted small pox. He returned to Berhampur to succumb only after a week, in the month of *Baisakha* on the auspicious day of *Akshay Trutiya.*

Kabisurya not only wrote in Oriya but also in Sanskrit, Urdu, Hindi and Telugu. He excelled in different forms of Oriya poetry like *Champu, Chautisa, Chaupadi,* etc. His songs, by and large, are about the love of Krishna and Radha, mainly in the romantic scale. But Baladeva's *Magnum Opus* in the field of songs in Orissa is the celebrated *Kishore Chandrananda Champu,* which comprises of a total of 34 songs. These are the favourites of the *gotipua* dancers and also for the modern day Odissi. The songs are in alphabetical order, covering the 34 consonants in the Oriya alphabet from *Ka* to *Kshya*, narrating the romantic love-play between Radha and Krishna. Another peculiar feature of each *Champu* was that all the lines of the lyric also started with the same consonant – a rather crafty composition of lyrics. Being a poet and musician at the same time, he also has specified the *raga* and *tala* for each *Champu.* For example, for the *Ka Champu*, he has specified *raga Saveri* and *tala Tripata* and for the last one (*Kshya Champu*) he has specified *raga Kedara* and *tala Tisra tripata.* As mentioned in the section on *gotipuas*, interpretation of *Champu* was a must for the *gotipuas* who sang and interpreted the lyrics. A very common song, popular in Odissi, is the *Bha Champu: Bhangi Chahan.* This particular song very popular among the *gotipuas*, was brought in to modern day Odissi. The translation by Late Dr. Mayadhar Mansinha, who took a lot of trouble to translate it for me as he was keen that the non-Oriya audience got the correct idea of the lyrics, is given at the end of the chapter.

Another composition of towering significance is his *Sarpa Janana-Badhila Janikshsyama* in *raga Kamodi.* Here the poet has literally accused Lord Jagannath of being a snake and puts forth several evidences in favour of it. At the end is an interesting *Bhanati* (dedication) where the lyrics imply that Lord Jagannath is worried that *Kabisurya* may let out this secret. Then *Kabisurya* makes the most touching deal:

> Don't worry Lord Jagannath, only you and I know that you are a snake and I will not let out this secret on one condition that when *Tarata* (Yama) comes to take me, you will liberate me from his door (meaning hell).

Apparently, during his short stay with the Raja, he used to go daily to the temple and sing (in a way rebuke) to Lord Jagannath for causing much misery to him through the *Sarpa Janana*. At a philosophical level, it is said that the song carries the concept of *bhakta adhina Bhagaban*. When *Kabisurya* threatens to let out the secret that Lord Jagannath is actually a snake out to cause harm in many ways, Lord Jagannath is worried that his *bhaktas* may not respect him anymore. He thus almost comes down to *Kabisurya's* level to make a deal. This is a song very close to the Oriya heart and most can sing it in the traditional tune which has come down from generation to generation. My paternal grand-mother used to make me sing this song to her everyday as my paternal grand-father's name Jagabandhu, often appears in the refrain.

GOPALKRUSHNA (1884-1861)

Gopalkrushna was the eldest son of Shri Banabasi Patnaik, the *Panjia Karana* (the one who is in-charge of the records like a gazetteer) of the Maharaja of Parlakhemundi. Thus, like *Kabisurya*, he also belonged to Ganjam district. Gopalkrushna belonged to a well-to-do family and was a devout *Vaishnava*. Gopalkrushna is the only poet in medieval Oriya literature to sing enchantingly of the naughty childhood of Krishna. Through many songs he has depicted Lord Krishna as a cowherd boy going to tend cattle in distant forests, causing much mental suffering to his mother Yasoda. He has also depicted Krishna's life from pre-adolescence, adolescence to romance period. His lyrics are known for their purity and sublimity of emotions expressed in the most natural way, without any ornamentation. It caught the imagination of people and his lyrics became popular both in northern and southern parts of Orissa. During Gopalkrushna's time, Paralakhemundi was under Madras Presidency and *gurus* from Andhra used to give lessons in music during this period. Therefore, many *ragas* and *talas* from Carnatic music has been recommended by him for his songs.

A characteristic feature of his songs is the ending "Maa". As a matter of fact, this word is taken as a clue to his lyrics. In comparison to those of *Kabisurya*, his lyrics are simple and sweet. The translation of the song *Shyamaku Juhara* (by Late Dr. Mayadhar Mansinha), is given at the end of this chapter as it used to be a very popular item for *abhinaya* in those days.

BANAMALI (1720-?)

As there were several writers by the name "Banamali" during the medieval period, it has been difficult to get details of Banamali Das Pattanaik whose poems enjoy immense popularity in music, dance and literature. However, it is believed that Banamali has given the clue to his ancestry in his *Ramachampu* where he describes himself as belonging to *Dolamandapa sahi* in Puri. He has said that he is the son of Hari Das, belonging to the *Karana* caste. He has mentioned that he enjoyed the patronage of Khurda Raja Birakishore Deva who reigned from 1736 to 1793 AD. This gives the indication that Banamali belonged to this period. According to Banamali, he wrote *Ramachampu* under the instructions from his *guru* in his dream, Late Shri Lakhsmana Talichho. It is believed that Lakhsmana Talichho was an expert in music and under his influence, Banamali started writing poems. Banamali himself was a musician and specified *ragas* and *talas* for many of his poems. Banamali also wrote *Sachitra Ramayana* which he dedicated to his father. Apparently, he was thirty years old when he completed this volume and based on this, it is computed that he was born sometime between 1720 to 1725.

Of Banamali, who unlike his two predecessors was a real *Vaishnavite sanyasi*, the songs are not as numerous as those of *Kabisurya* or Gopalkrushna but are extremely popular. His speciality lies in the simplicity of lyrics which are forthright and throb with sincerity of a true zealot and touches the soul. The song *Dinena Dakibu Radhika Boli* is part of a ritual song during *chapa* whose translation is given below.

SPORTS OF KRISHNA

Darling, this is sweet spring-time, when soft *Malaya* breeze blows,
bringing fragrance of gently trembling creepers of clove
and the groves echo with the hum of bees and songs of cuckoos.
And in this budding spring-time, unkind to those separated from dear ones,
Krishna dallies elsewhere with sweet young things.

When women deeply desiring the pleasures of love
but, deserted, bewail their lot,
when the *Bakula* trees are covered with fragrant flowers,
and the flowers, in turn, are covered with the bees,
Krishna chooses to have a gay time at this hour with sweet young things,
When the delicate leaves of the *Tamala* emit fragrance like musk
and red curved Palasa flowers look like nails of Cupid
that delight in tearing the hearts of youth,
it is in such fine spring time that
Krishna chooses to have a gay time with sweet young things.

When the *Nagakeshara* trees with their long golden flowers look like sceptres of Kama, the Love God
and Patali trees, their flowers having been thickly covered by bees,
look like Kama's quivers, it is in such fine spring-time that
Krishna chooses to have a gay time with sweet young things.

When Karuna plants, observing how the whole creation has lost all sense of delicacy,
because of the sweet season, smile as it were through their blossoms,
and, all around the tapering ends of *Ketaki* flowers stand arrayed,
like *Cupid's* spears to stab the hearts of those
separated from their dear ones, it is in such fine spring-time that
Krishna chooses to have a gay time with sweet young things.
when the air is delicately scented with the fragrance of Madhavi flowers,
and heavy with those of *Malati* and *Jasmine*,
the time when the minds of even ascetics go astray,
but the time which is the natural friend of youth,
Krishna chooses to have a gay time with sweet young things.

When this *Vrinda* forest, whose fringe is sanctified by the holy steam of the Yamuna,
where mango trees, embraced by many a creeper, express their ecstasy,
as it were, in their lovely blossoms, it is in such fine spring-time, that
Krishna chooses to have a gay time with sweet young things.

Describing the fine spring-time, with its concomitant feelings of love,
this song of Jayadeva brings to mind the memory of Krishna's holy feet.

(Translated by Dr. Mayadhar Mansinha from Canto I
of the *Gita Govinda* by Jayadeva).

RADHA'S CONFIDANTE TO KRISHNA

(about Radha's desperate condition in love)

Spurning delights of moonlight and sandal paste
she, the desperate one, deems even the southern breeze as poison,
coming as it does from the *Malaya* Hill, infested with snakes.
O Krishna, my friend Radha is so desperately sad without you
that as her only refuge from the arrows of Cupid
she seems already lost in you, in imagination (Refrain)

And imagining you to be already united with her
and that you too are a target of Kama's attacks,
she covers her breasts with lotus leaves as though to protect you.
The bed of flowers that was meant for pleasures
is now turned into one of arrows
and she, sleeping on that, is undergoing a penance,
as it were, for the ultimate blessing of your embrace.
Her lotus face is now darkened with a cloud of sorrow
and the moon of her face is shedding as it were streams of nectar.
In the shape of tears, bitten with Rahu's awesome teeth.

Along, she paints your likeness in musk
like an imitation of Kama, placing the picture of *Makara* below it.
And putting mango blossoms in your hands for the arrows of Cupid.

And she makes obeisance to you.
These are the words that are ever on her lips:
"O Krishna, I lie prostrate before you:
as you continue to be unkind to me,
the Moon, supposed to be the repository of ambrosia,
is ever scorching my body and my soul."

And thinking again that you are beyond her expectations in spite of all these sufferings,
she sometimes loses her mental balance,
(and cries and laughs) or behaves as if nothing had happened.

If you, oh Reader, would like to have more mental entertainment
out of the poet Jayadeva's songs, then listen, please,
to the words of Radha's friend as she describes
the pitiful condition of cowherd girls in separation from Krishna.

(Translated by Dr. Mayadhar Mansinha from Canto IV
of Jayadeva's *Gita Govinda*)

CONFIDANTE DESCRIBES TO KRISHNA, RADHA'S EXPECTANT WAITING FOR HIM

Oh Lord Krishna, wistfully waiting for you,
Radha gets despondent as she visualises you everywhere
sucking sweet honey off the lips of women.

Desperate, she ventures out of the house to have a
tryst with you, but falls down on the ground after
only a few steps, unsteady under the burden of her
agitated emotions.

Constantly glancing over her make-ups, she so gets immersed in thoughts of you, that lost to all realities, she often imagines "I too am he."
Again and again she queries her friends, "why is He not coming soon to me?"

Her friends, taking off the bejewelled bangles, have decorated her hands with stalks of white lotus to cool her hot emotions. That the poor thing is still surviving is for only the last lingering hope of a union with you.

So lost is the poor darling to all senses, that she even runs to kiss and embrace the encompassing darkness of the night which reminds her of you.

The more you delay your visit, the more she loses all
sense of dignity and starts moaning and weeping.

Let this lyric by poet Jayadeva generate pleasure
in the hearts of understanding persons.

(Translated by Dr. Mayadhar Mansinha from Canto VI
of Jayadeva's *Gita Govinda*)

KRISHNA PROVES FALSE

He did not turn up, though the appointed time has long passed.
Beguiled as I was by the words of friends,
I now realize the worthlessness of my youth and beauty,
who shall be my refuge now? (Refrain)

He, to follow whom I have roamed every part of this
deep forest at night, has left my heart
as smitten by Cupid's arrows as before.

Death shall be my only refuge now. How should I
go on suffering such pangs of separation any longer,
as I have been doing so far, in ignorance?

Although this charming spring night is so painful to me,
some other blessed woman is, perhaps,
even now, enjoying *Hari's* love.

I hate even all these bejewelled bracelets of mine,
as they too have absorbed the heat of my mad love for Krishna.

And even this flower garland over my flower-delicate body
is hurting my heart.
I roam about among the thorny canes of the forest
looking for *Hari*, but he thinks so little of me.

Let these words of the poet Jayadeva stay in the hearts
of men like a sweet young girl, full of charms.

(Translated by Dr. Mayadhar Mansinha from Canto VII
of Jayadeva's *Gita Govinda*)

LALITA, THE CONFIDANTE SPEAKS

(to Radha, when she sees Krishna from a distance, at her first tryst)

Look Darling, at those eyebrows of His
that wave like a black serpent.
It is worth one's whole existence to have a glimpse of such beauty.

But lest, Darling, you lose your balance
in the mad desire for instant union with such beauty
you had better steady yourself,
encircling me with your delicate arms
and fixing firmly your lotus feet on the ground.

Beautifier of this world as you are, mark, Darling.,
the unparalleled grace of His moon-like face
with the paint of *Gorachana* on His forehead,
and the ever moving crown of peacock feather's just above.

(Translated by Dr. Mayadhar Mansinha from the first
two stanzas of *Kabisurya* Baladeva Ratha's famous
"*Kishorechandrananda Champu*" (*Bhangi Chahan*).

RADHA TO HER CONFIDANTE

(at the latter's suggestion of a possible liaison with Krishna)

Goodbye, Darling, to Shyama, goodbye to His romances
Only a woman whose heart is made of steel
could desire for an affair with Him (Refrain)

Isn't He the same about whom the drum of gossip is ever beaten in the whole of this *Vraja*
in connection with that woman *Chandravali*?

And they say He kidnaps any he fancies from among
the cowherd girls while on their way to Mathura to sell curds
and takes her to one of the caves of *Govardhana* Hill.

If I ever came within the clutches of such as He,
would it not be like getting drowned in a sea of misery?
And could I look people in the face as long as I live?

Once, indeed, I caught a glimpse of Him from a distance
as He stood under a *Nipa* tree,
and as He was offering me a necklace.
I ran away for the life of me.

But, says *Gopalakrushna*, My Lady,
it is for you only that the Prince of *Vraja*
has turned into a mere cattle-tender.

(Translated by Dr. Mayadhar Mansinha from an Oriya poem,
"*Shyamaku juhara*" by Gopalakrushna)

RADHA'S APPEAL TO THE FLUTE

I prostrate myself, and appeal to you, Oh Krishna's flute,
Not to call, please, 'Radha' on any day (Refrain)

He, your owner, is a cowherd boy, and I a princess:
It is, indeed, you, Flute, that has made us know each other
How did you, Flute, pick me out of all the girls,
The shiest of all, who stealthily comes and goes,
and never without companions if ever she goes out?

Descended as you are from a thorny piece of bamboo,
Your sound, likewise, is sharply piercing.

And if, perchance, someone wrenched you out of Krishna's palms
and put you in mine, I would fain float you down Yamuna's current.

You are impertinent enough a mere flute
To aspire to lead virtuous women astray:
I appeal to you, therefore, with folded hands,
Not to utter my name ever again, ever again.

(Translated by Dr. Mayadhar Mansinha from an oriya poem,
"*Dinena dakibu Radhika boli*" by Banamali).

REFERENCES

Champu-Swaralipi, (in Oriya) 1963. Sangeet Natak Akademi, Bhubaneswar.

Das, Brahmananda, 1964. *Odisare' Sangeetara Parampara, Jaha Odisara taha Odissi* (in Oriya).

Das, Dasarathi, 1987. *Kavisurya Baladeva Rath*, Sahitya Akademi, New Delhi.

Das, Ramahari, 1986. *Odissi Sangeeta Parampara*, Keteka Sangeetkara O' Sangeetakruti, Utkal Pathak Sansad, Cuttack.

Fabri, Charles, 1961. "Introduction: Brochure for the Performance of Priyambada Mohanty", *The Little Theater Group*, Delhi.

Hansadwani, Utkal Sangeet Mahavidyalaya, Bhubaneswar.

Kabichandra Kalicharan Patnaik. 1981. *Amara Sangeeta Dhara* (in Oriya), Sathi Mahal, Cuttack.

Kabisurya Geetabali (in Oriya), (edited by *Kabichandra* Kalicharan Patnaik), published by Jagannath Rath, Cuttack.

Khokar, Mohan, 1985. "My Initiation, Souvenir of Angahar Festival", New Delhi.

Mahapatra, K., 1973. *Shri Jayadeva O' Shri Gitagovinda* (in Oriya), Grantha Karta, Bhubaneswar.

Rahman, Indrani, 1993. "Revival of Odissi Dance", *Tahiya*, Srikhsetra Kala Prakashika, Second Jugapurti Utsab, Puri.

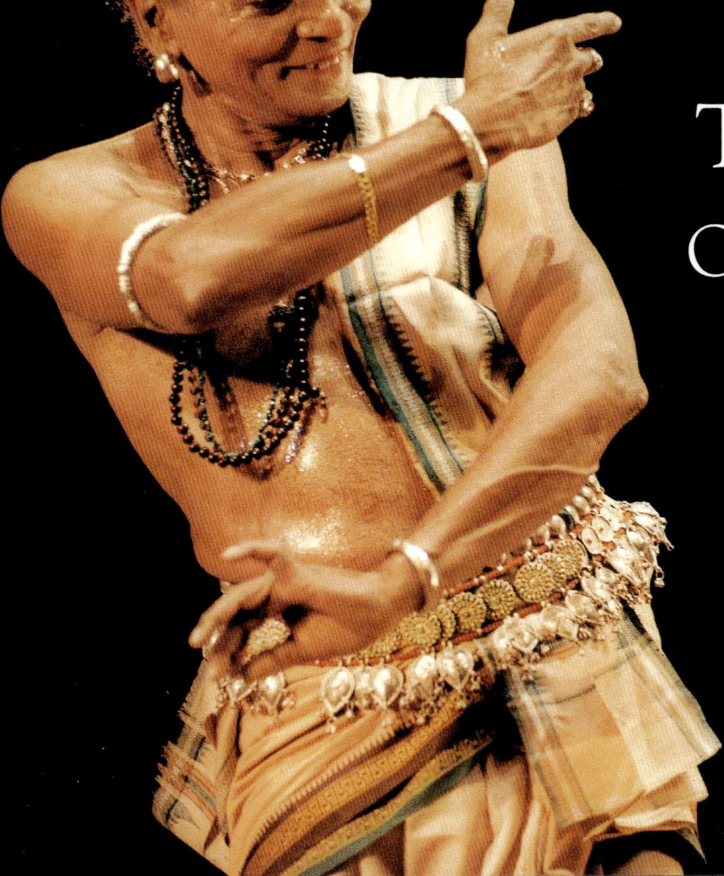

The Architects of Odissi Dance – Gurus

4

Odissi dance as it is known today, owes its existence to the outstanding *gurus* who not only perpetuated but also developed the tradition to the codified and sophisticated present form. The origin may have much to do with the *mahari* and *gotipua* systems but the development of its present form depended heavily on the popular *Rasa Leela* and *Jatra* tradition during the early part of the 19th century. A few outstanding persons who took up dance and music purely due to their love for it and at times against the wishes of their parents, in retrospect are the real architects who laid the foundation for the modern day Odissi dance and music. We can divide them broadly into two generations – the early generation and the later involving those upto 1950's and those after 1950's, respectively. During the early period, although, many people were practising dance and music with their increasing popularity, two people deserve mention who played an active role in training the next generation of dancers and musicians – *Singhari* Shayamasunder Kar and Shri Durllav Chandra Singh. Similarly, during the latter period, with music and dance being accepted by the society and a demand for tutors in the families of educataed class, more people took up teaching music and dance. However, three people had considerable influence in the shaping of dance into three distinctive styles within the framework of Odissi. They are Pankaj Charan Das, Kelucharan Mohapatra and Debaprasad Das. I consider them as the trinity of Odissi (Mohanty-Hejmadi, 1990). In this chapter, I deem it fit to give a glimpse into these assorted group of people who established a *guru parampara* for Odissi which was completely non-existent earlier.

SINGHARI SHYAMASUNDER KAR

The doyen of Odissi music and dance, Shyamasunder belonged to the traditional *Singhari* family permanently attached to the Jagannath temple. Son of Shri Gobinda Chandra Kar and Shrimati Padmabati, Shyamasunder was born on March 4,1908 in *Manikarnika Sahi* in Puri. Although he was born into a *Singhari* family who were in-charge of the rituals associated with decorating Lord Jagannath in the evening (known as the *Bada Singhara Vesha*), his real love was music. He was attracted to music from his very

FACING PAGE :
Bandha solo.

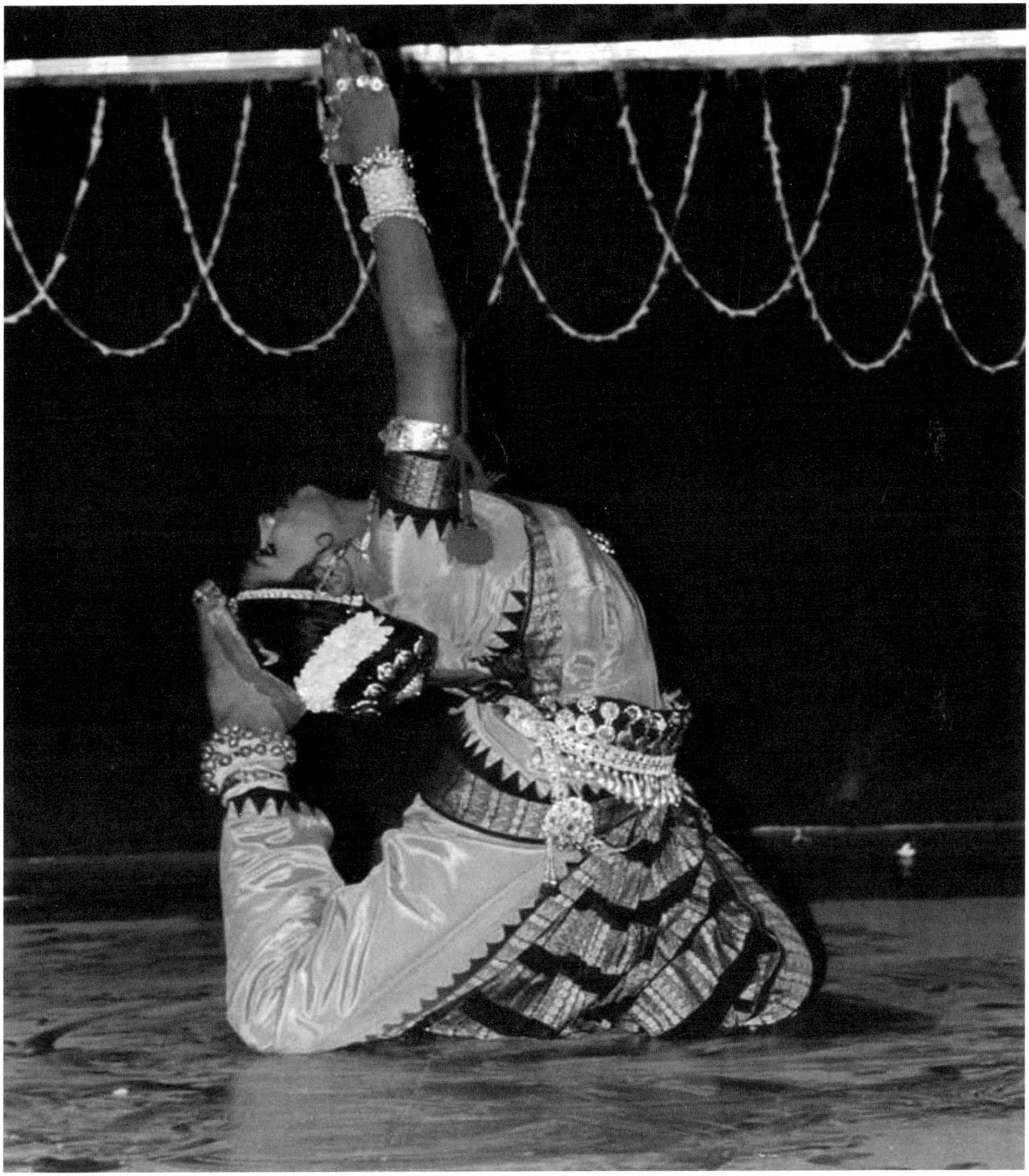

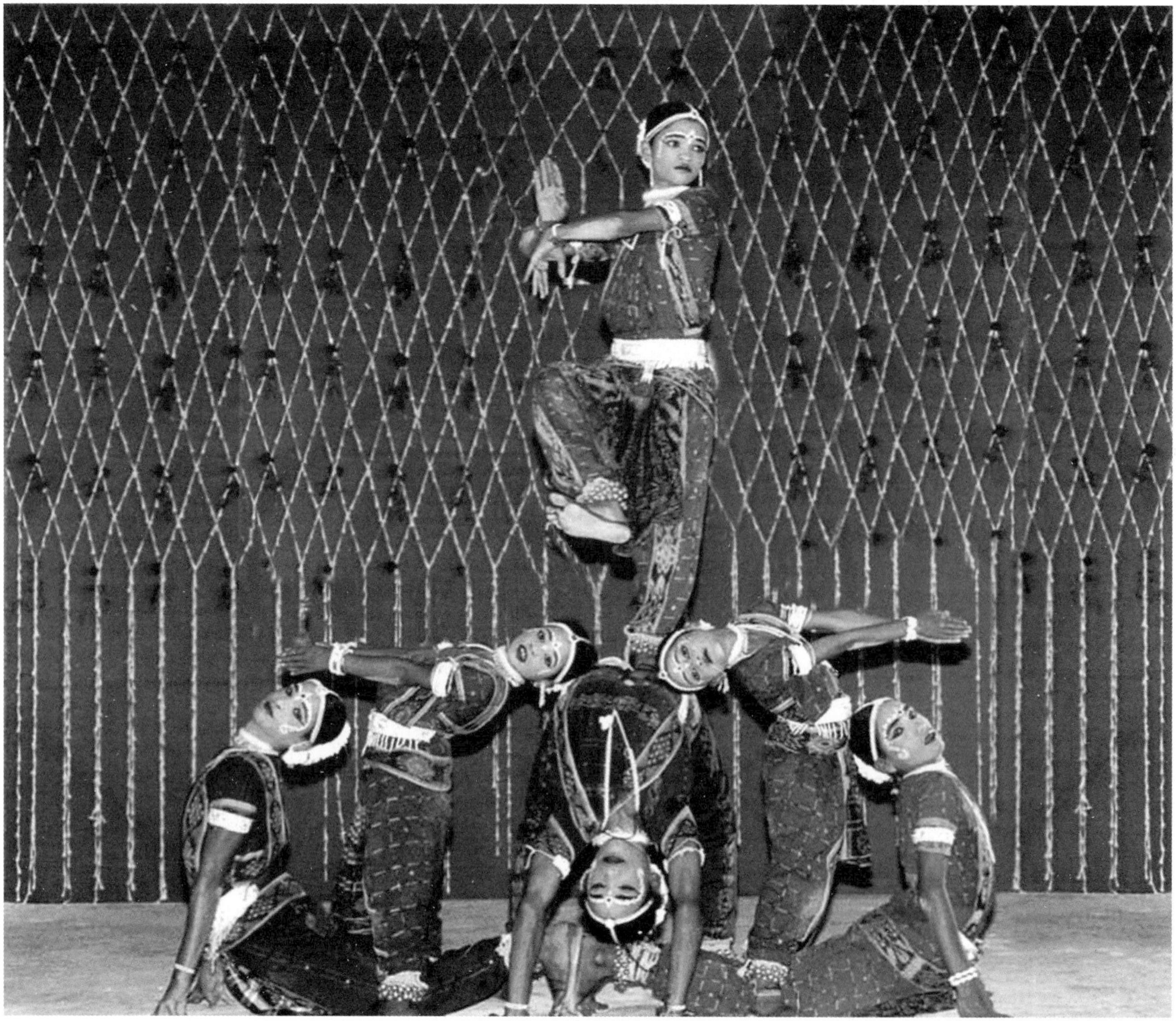

Bandha group formations.

childhood when Puri was pulsating with cultural activities. He used to sneak out of the house at night to see theatre, *Suanga*, *Ram Leela* and *Ras Leela*, etc. which was a daily affair in Puri. Although he received his formal education in a Sanskrit toll (school), he by his own efforts learnt Odissi music (both vocal and *mardal)* from the famous musicians, namely Gadi Jagannath

Pratihari, Kalpataru Naik, Andha Managobinda Mohanty, Chintamani Mishra and Harihar Rayaguru. He also took advantage of the visits of Hindustani *ustads* to Puri for performances. He gained thorough knowledge of *Dhrupad* and *Kheyal* from Balabanta Rao, Brahmanand Goswami, Pandit Ramachandra and Jashobanta Mule to name a few. With training in both Odissi and Hindusthani music, he dominated the field of music and dance from pre-Independence to post-Independence period. As a musician, he was much in demand in all festivals in Orissa and soon reached a legendary status as *Singhari*. He was a regular artiste of All India Radio, Calcutta, initially and then Cuttack after its establishment in 1948. He used to impart lessons in Odissi music in all the leading institutions of Cuttack and Puri, and finally the Utkal Sangeet Mahavidyalaya when it was established in 1964, where he continued to train next generations of Odissi musicians both in vocal and instrumental *(mardala)* music until his sad demise on March 16, 1975.

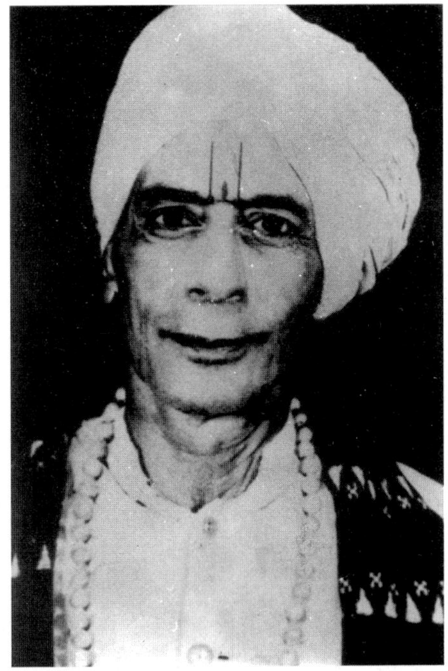

Singhari Shyamasunder Kar.

Singhari also used to visit the *akhadagharas* (literally meaning gymnasium for acrobatics which were also the seats of learning for music and dance exclusively for men) in Puri where he learnt dances related to *gotipua* and *sahi jatra* traditions. He had the additional advantage of seeing the rituals of *maharis* during the *Badasinghara Vesha* in the Jagannath temple. As a matter of fact he also trained a few *maharis* in music. Outstanding amongst them was *mahari* Parasamani who became an artiste of All India Radio in 1940's. In Utkal Sangeet Samaj, at Cuttack, in addition to the lessons in music, he used to teach Odissi dance to a few of us. He was the consultant for music and dance for all the theatres in Cuttack. According to Durllav Chandra Singh, who acted as Jayadeva, *Singhari* contributed significantly to the music and dance compositions for Jayadeva drama written and produced by Late *Kabichandra* Kalicharan Patnaik, under the auspices of Orissa theatres in the early 1940's. The same tunes and *bols* (rhythmic syllables) are still used in Odissi music and dance today. *Singhari* is the only musician from Orissa who had the unique privilege of giving an Odissi recital in the All India Music Festival in New Delhi, on March 27, 1954, rendering vocal music and playing the *mardala*. *Singhari* not only dominated but also developed Odissi music to what it is today. What is interesting is that while regularly conducting his *Singhari seva*, he used to act and dance as Parasuram for *Harchandi sahi* during the the *Sahi jatra*, in the month of *Chaitra*. In addition, he could train and leave a strong line of musicians for perpetuating the art for the future generations. He received many prestigious awards from Utkal Sahitya Samaj, Prajatantra Prachar Samiti, Bhanja Sahitya Samaj, etc., and Orissa Sangeet Natak Akademi Award in 1972. He also was honoured with several titles, namely *Gayakaratna, Sangitacharya, Srikshetraratna* and *Sangitabisari* for his outstanding contribution to music. Taking music as his mission in life, he wrote two books, "Srikshetra Bhajanamala" and "Raganamabrutya". He was the technical consultant and provided the *talas* and *bols* for the booklet on Odissi dance (Patnaik, undated). In a rare gesture, he donated his own house to Shyamasunder Sangeet Mahavidyalaya which he had established in Puri to impart training in music.

Shri Durllav Chandra Singh, 2002.

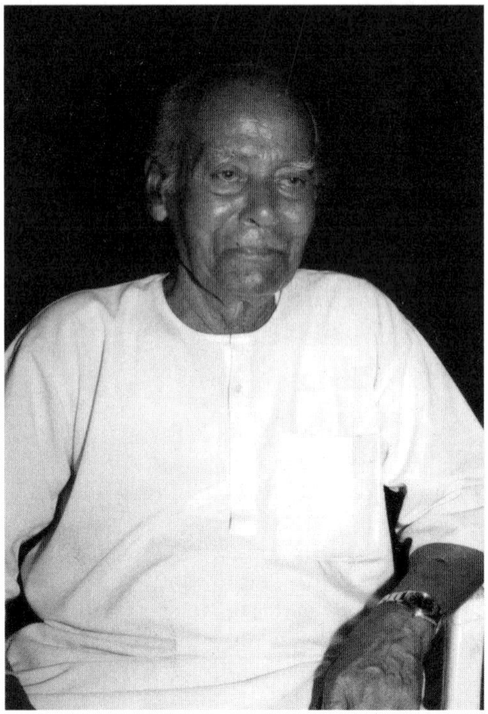

DURLLAV CHANDRA SINGH

A legendary figure in theatre of Orissa, Durllav Chandra Singh was born in Nimapara in Puri district, in 1917. His father, Anandachandra Singh, was famous as the *ustad* who used to impart training in acting, could play the *mardal* and violin with exceptional skill, and also was a director for dance. Naturally, all this rubbed off well on young Durllav. He was trained in dance, music and acting, by his father. He had to discontinue his formal education due to financial difficulties and joined the *jatra* at a very tender age. Durllav Chandra grew up in a very critical period when *jatra* underwent modernisation. This was also the period when *Rasa Leela* troupes emerged in the cultural scene. Durllav Chandra joined the *Rasa Leela* party of Late *Kabichandra* Kalicharan Patnaik in 1929 and from him got further training in dance, music and acting. Ultimately *Kabichandra* converted his *Rasa* troupe to Odissa theatre in 1940 to promote theatre in Orissa. Almost all the senior dancers, musicians and actors of Orissa were members of Orissa theatres who were trained by Late *Kabichandra* Kalicharan Patnaik.

Durllav Chandra not only excelled in acting but also contributed significantly to the music and dance compositions in Orissa theatre. He is still remembered for his outstanding performance as Jayadeva, a drama on the life of Jayadeva written and produced by *Kabichandra*. It is noteworthy that *Kabichandra* and Durllav Chandra, with the help of *Singhari*, had composed a *Mahari* dance for Hemalata who danced in front of a replica of *Kalaghata Dwara* of Jagannath temple in the play. This is of historical importance and perhaps the only attempt in using a *mahari* dance in theatre. However, time came when *Kabichandra* could not sustain Orissa theatre and had to dismantle his group, which eventually led to the migration of seasoned artistes to other theatres. Durllav Chandra joined the Annapurna "B" group where, in addition to acting, he was involved in direction and composition of dance and music as and when necessary. When Annapurna "B" group also dismantled in 1955, he joined Annapurna "A" group and continues to be associated with it till today. It is rewarding to see Durllav Babu still acting in occasional productions of Annapurna "A" group at the ripe old age of 85.

His dance training in his childhood, during his *Ras Leela* days and under *Kabichandra*, gave him an edge over other contemporary dance teachers associated with theatre. He has contributed significantly to the choreography as well as musical accompaniment for different items as documented by Citaristi (2001). Amongst his many students, the most famous are Kelucharan Mohapatra and Shrimati Laxmipriya Devi.

Durllav Babu has received several prestigious awards, namely Bishubamilana Puraskara of Prajatantra Prachar Samiti, Orissa Cultural Association, Ganakabi Shruti Samsad, Utkal Pathak Samsad, Guru Kelucharan Mohapatra Samman, Orissa Sangeet Natak Akademi, in 1975, Central Sangeet Natak Akademi, in 2003 and the Upendra Bhanja Samman, the highest award of Orissa Sangeet Natak Akademi for his lifetime contribution in 1995. He has chronicled his life and times in his autobiography (Singh, 1988).

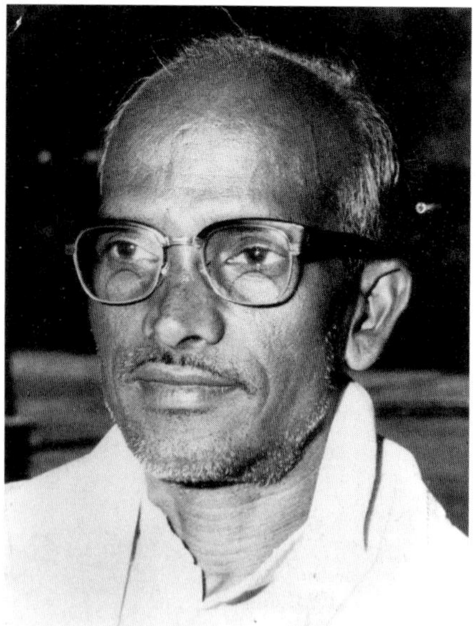

Guru Pankaj Charan Das, 1971 (courtesy: Central Sangeet Natak Akademi, New Delhi).

PANKAJ CHARAN DAS

Pankaj Charan Das of Puri belongs to a *madeli* family attached to the Jagannath temple. The *madelis* provide *mardal* or drum accompaniment to the *maharis*. He is the son of Kshetramani and Dharme Das, a policeman. Dharme Das died before Pankaj Charan was born and he was brought up by his mother in very difficult circumstances. Kshetramani and young Pankaj Charan lived with Fakira *mahari* and his aunt, Ratnaprava *mahari* and therefore, he was exposed to music and dance from his very infancy. According to him, he was consciously attracted to dance and music in his early childhood. He could easily repeat the dances and music practiced by the *maharis* at home so much so that young *mahari* trainees were often asked to "sing and dance like Pankaj" by the senior *maharis* teaching them. In the evenings, he used to go to an *akhadaghara*. Here he was exposed to the more vigorous singing and dancing style of the *gotipuas*. Thus, he acquired a sound background in both the *mahari* and *gotipua* styles of dance and music. Therefore, his choreography has a range of items, some of which are in the typically demure lyrical style of the *maharis* and some in the more perky effervescent style of the *gotipuas*.

Unconsciously absorbing the art initially in a *mahari* family – chiefly from his aunt Ratraprava – and then consciously seeking training in an *akhadaghara*, and still later from Ranganath Dev Goswami and Bhikari Charan Dalei of *Ras Leela* troupes, Pankaj Charan grew into a fine performer. As a boy, he used to participate in dance, music and plays at school. Later he started giving occasional performances at the Hajuri theatre in Puri. During his training in *akhadaghara* he learnt the two most popular virtuoso items of the *gotipua* repertoire – the acrobatic *bandha nrutya* and the skilful *thali nrutya*. A big attraction in those days was the *thali nrutya* competition between him and Bhagi *Suara* where they tried to outdo each other by impromptu variations in the maneuver of the *thalis* in hand and foot, much to the delight of the audience. Of course, it was not possible for him to earn his living only by giving performances. It is noteworthy to mention that this great *guru* earned his living first as a hawker of *pan* and a *pan* seller in a betel shop and later as a part-time peon in Puri.

FACING PAGE : *Guru Pankaj Charan Das with Ahalya.*

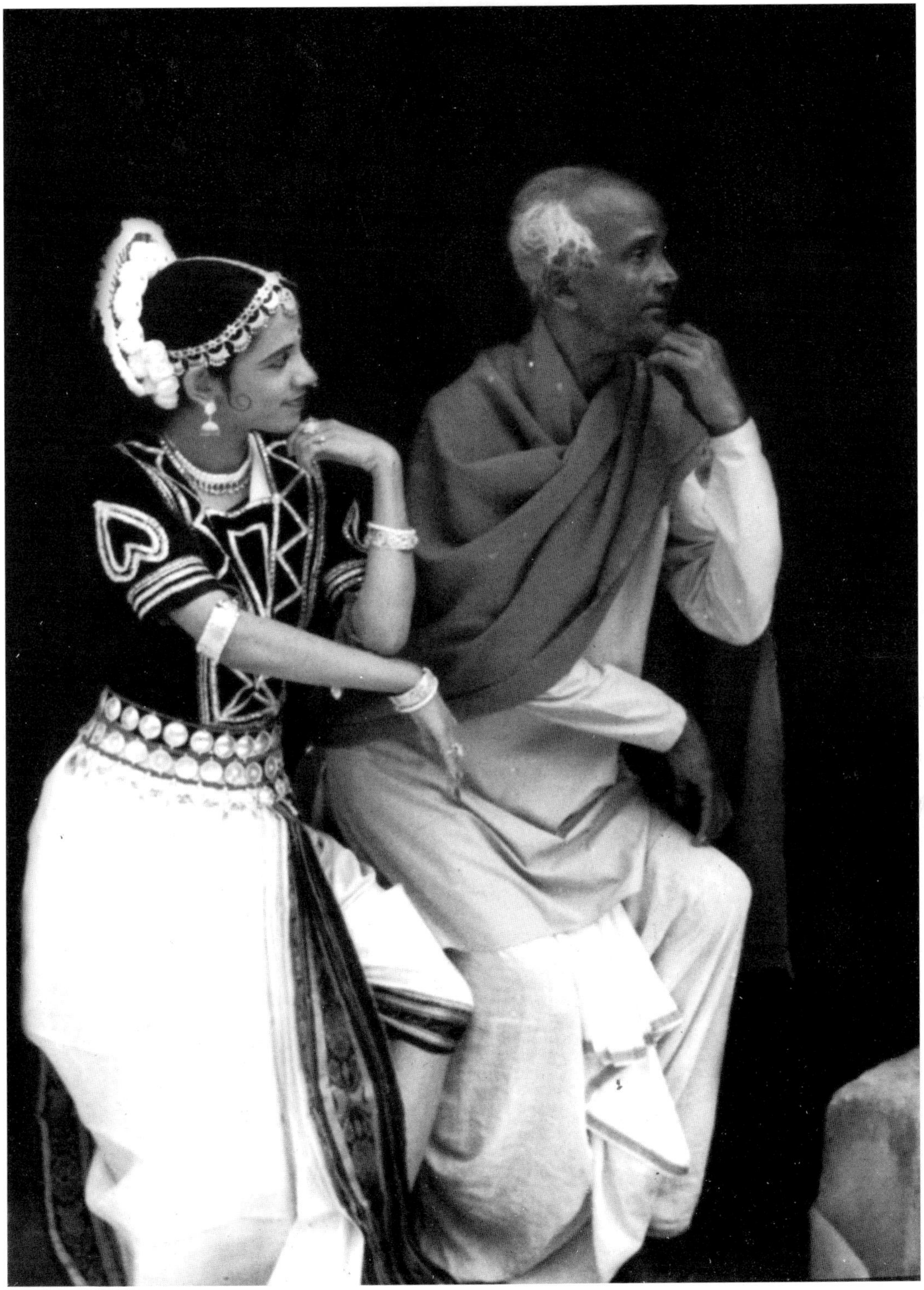

The turning point in his life came when he joined New theatres and travelled all over Orissa singing, dancing and acting. He began his career as a dance teacher at Annapurna theatre in Cuttack. He also choreographed dances for the plays staged in the theatre. A fact of historical significance for Odissi is that during this period he taught dance to the husband-wife team of Kelucharan and Laxmipriya Mohapatra who were then young artistes employed in the Annapurna theatre. He choreographed several episodes from mythology. In the *Bhasmasura* episode, he acted as *Bhasmasura* with Kelucharan and Laxmipriya playing *Nataraj* and *Mohini*, respectively. He also choreographed the *dashavatara* with Durllav Singh as a duet for Kelucharan and Laxmipriya. This was around the time when he and his colleagues were exposed to the book by Projesh Banerjee "Dances of India" and became aware of the use of *mudras* to express the meaning of words. For the first time in the Odissi tradition, he and Durllav Babu used different *mudras* for each of the *avataras*. I consider *dashavatara* the first work of modern choreography in Odissi; it was a landmark which started a new trend in Odissi dance which till then had employed traditional *mudras* (*Parijas*) in a limited way. Pankaj Charan was in of Annapurna theatre from 1944 to 1949.

The early 50's saw a change in the the attitude towards music and dance in Orissa, specially in Cuttack which was the centre of all cultural activities. Dance teachers started earning a living independently by teaching dance, mainly in music schools. Educated people were also willing to train their daughters in music and dance, and this opened up to *gurus* the avenue for private tuition. Around this time, Pankaj Charan also began to be noticed by presenting his work outside Annapurna theatre. His repertoire included, among other modified traditional items, the popular *bandha nrutya, thali nrutya* and *dashavatara.*

After Priyambada's performance in Delhi, in 1954, we were invited to participate in the National Dance Festival there in 1955. Pankaj Charan and Kelucharan choreographed the dance drama *Sakhigopal* for the festival with lyrics by *Kabichandra* Kalicharan Patnaik, which earned much acclaim from by the critics. Subsequently, he continued to teach dance and enrich the Odissi repertoire with new choreography. With Odissi gaining momentum, he was invited to teach Yamini Krishnamurthy and Sumathi Kaushal. This gave him the exposure to other forms of classical dance.

Being the most innovative and adventurous of the three *gurus*, Pankaj Charan started experimenting with *Mangalacharan*. Deviating from the custom of beginning a performance with *Ganesh Vandana*, he introduced a *manchapravesha* to Shankaracharya's *Jagannathstaka – Jagannath Swami Nayanapathagami*. According to Hindu tradition as well as the Odissi tradition, or more specifically the *gotipua* tradition, Lord Ganesha, being *Vighnaraja*, was to be worshipped first among all other deities! But innovations like this have marked the expansion and evolution of Odissi throughout history. As a choreographer, Pankaj Charan excelled in solo as well as group items or *mela nrutya*.

Pankaj Charan joined Utkal Sangeet Mahavidyalaya in Bhubaneswar in the early 60's and his tenure there can be considered the most productive part of his career. He trained several generations of dancers at the Mahavidyalaya, including most of the young dance *gurus* of today. His items bear the stamp of the *mahari* tradition distinguished by *atibhanga* and peculiar flip-flop walks. Some of his popular items are the *pallavis* in *ragas Shankarbharana, Arabhi, Kalyan, Deshakhya*, etc. His *sthayi* is sculpturesque in which the transitions are very smooth, with assertive *chauka* punctuations. In *abhinaya*, besides the usual *ashtapadi* pieces of Jayadeva like *dashavatar* and *Badasi Yadi*, he has choreographed some really perky *gotipua*-style pieces like *Radharani Songé Naché* or *Nachanti Rangé Srihari*, besides a series of thematic dances on the *Panchakanyas – Ahalya, Draupadi, Kunti, Tara* and *Mandodari*. His *pallavi* "*Gatibbilasa*" is an innovative piece. The use of animated movements to *tala* patterns to the traditional *pallavi* tune interspersed with Sanskrit *shloka* for each *gati* makes it an item for connoisseur. He loves to use Oriya lyrics – sometimes by famous authors like *Tuhima Janamabhumi* in praise of Mother India by Bhaktakabi Madhusudan Rao and sometimes by anonymous poets for his dance dramas like *mela nrutyas*. His *piéce de resistence* is, of course, the spectacular *Glani Samhara* based on the stories of *dashavatara*. Pankaj Charan started the practice of casting male dancers in male roles, imparting a special vigour to his choreography. It is an interesting feature in his choreography that once he stages a new composition, it catches the imagination of dancers. For example, after I performed the *Nabadurga* for my award ceremony by Central Sangeet Natak Akademi, in 1986, it spread like wildfire.

Nabadurga was choreographed by him, based on Oriya lyrics he picked up from a booklet on the footpath. Even famous disciples of other *gurus* are doing this now as a solo, as a duet or a group piece. His *Madhurastaka* is beginning to get very popular. Shri Harihara Panda has composed music for most of his pieces.

Guru Shri Das has the unique distinction of receiving the Orissa Sangeet Natak Akademi award in the field of dance and the Upendra Bhanja Samman, in 1970 and 1992, respectively (both in the first year of their institution). He has also received the Central Sangeet Natak Akademi Award, the Orissa Governor's Plaque and Padmashri for his contribution to Odissi.

KELUCHARAN MOHAPATRA

Kelucharan Mohapatra is now a legendary figure in the field of dance in India. He too had a humble beginning, was brought up in penurious circumstances in a *chitrakara* family in Raghurajpur, in Puri district. Son of Chintamani and Siri Nani, he was born in 1926. He was exposed to music from his infancy as his father was a proficient *khola* player. Kelucharan learnt to play the *khola* from his father which proved very valuable to him later as a dance teacher and *pakhawaj* player. His mastery over *tala* and his skill as a *pakhawaj* player has given him an advantage over other contemporary *gurus*.

Like other young boys in those days with an aptitude for music and dance, Kelucharan joined a *Ras Leela* troupe, one headed by the famous Guru Mohansunder Dev Goswami. Here he learnt acting, mime, dance, singing as well as make-up and stagecraft. He was with the troupe for 12 years. After leaving the troupe, he lived in dire poverty; it is again humbling to know that he worked for about a year doing odd jobs like rolling *bidis*, working as a labourer in betel farms and construction works.

Life took a better turn when he was hired by the Orissa theatre of *Kavichandra* Kalicharan Patnaik on a salary of seven rupees a month. His

FACING PAGE : *Guru Kelucharan Mahapatra.*

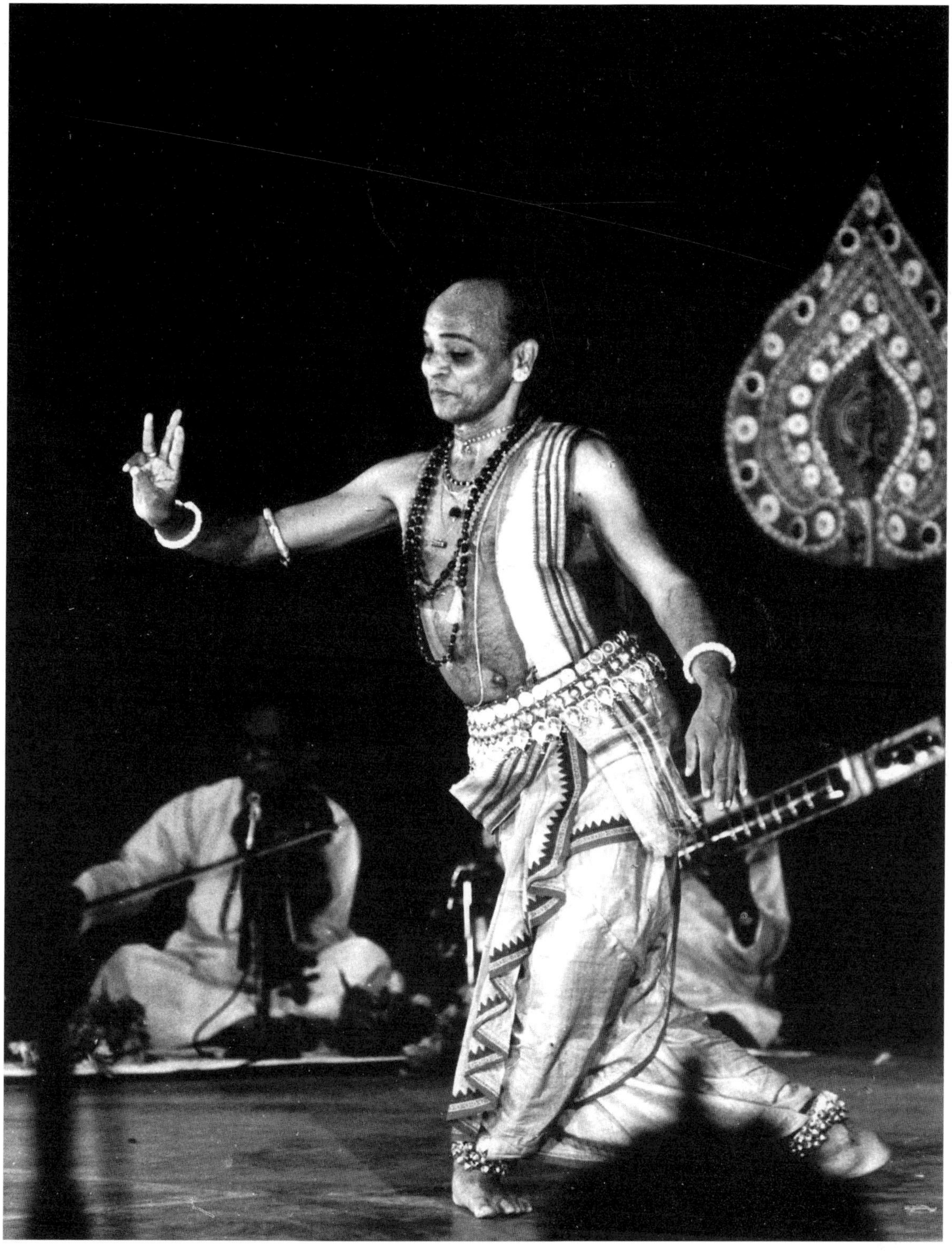

job was to help in stage work besides acting and playing percussion instruments. During this period, he received further training in *khola* from Agadhu Moharana, in *tabla* from the late Kshetramohan Kar and Harihar Rao. He then joined Annapurna theatre – a turning point in his career as a dancer. Pankaj Charan Das (whom he affectionately calls *Dada*) had, by then, already joined the Annapurna theatre. Trained by him and Durllav Chandra, Kelucharan excelled in the role of *Nataraja* in the composition on *Bhasmasura*. Laxmipriya, who was later to be his wife, acted as *Mohini* in this production. He also performed *dashavatara* with Laxmipriya which was choreographed by Durllav Chandra and Pankaj Charan.

After working for about five years with Annapurna theatre, Kelucharan and his wife Laxmipriya went to Puri and stayed there for a couple of years. At the age of 30, he joined the newly-established Kalavikash Kendra of Cuttack. It was here that he firmly established himself as a dance teacher, *pakhawaj* player and choreographer. He trained a group of young dancers at the Kendra some of whom are our present-day teachers. He also choreographed a number of dance dramas – *Shakuntala, Gita Govinda, Meghaduta, Urvashi, Champu*, etc. After working at Kalavikash Kendra for 15 years, he decided to leave the institution mainly to devote more time to choreography and to train some leading dancers including Sanjukta Mishra (Panigrahi), Sonal Mansingh and Kumkum Mohanty. He excelled in choreography and carved a niche for himself with his choreography of *astapadis* from Jayadeva's *Gita Govinda*. He worked closely with Bhubaneswar Mishra who set to music many of his *pallavis* which are notable items in the Odissi repertoire today (*Kalyan, Arabhi, Sankarabharana, Mohana, Khamaj, Bilahari*, etc). He has choreographed the largest number of items in Odissi and has considerably enriched its repertoire. His *batu* has the stamp of exactitude and a sculptural quality, his *pallavis* are woven-in with complex *tala* patterns, his *abhinayas* are extremely well balanced. Kelucharan has inspired dancers all over India to take up Odissi. The demand led to the establishment of training centres by him in Calcutta and the National Centre for the Performing Arts in Bombay.

A legend in his lifetime, Kelucharan has received honours and distinctions from many quarters. He received the Central Sangeet Natak Akademi Award

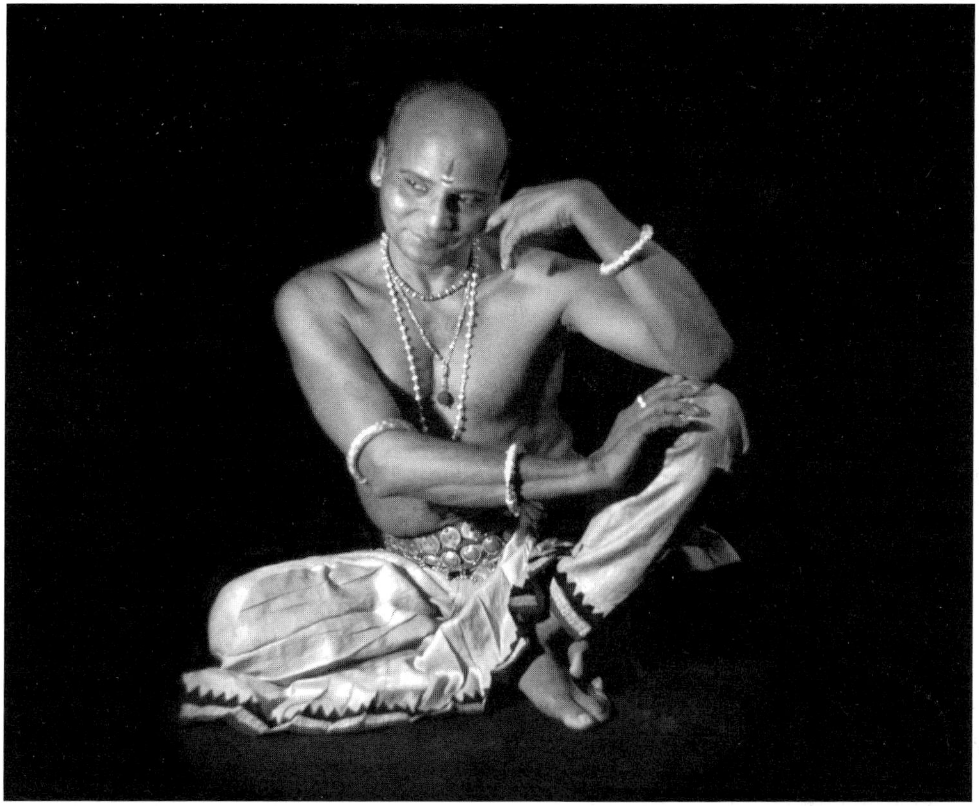

Guru Kelucharan Mahapatra (courtesy: Ratikanta Mahapatra).

and Fellowship in 1966 and 1987, respectively; the Padmashri, Padmabhushan and Padmavibhushan in 1972, 1989 and 2000, respectively; and the Kalidas Samman in 1989. He is also a recipient of the ITC Award from Sangeet Research Akademi, Calcutta, 1982. In addition, he received the Upendra Bhanja Award for his life time contribution to dance in 2000. He has also received an honorary doctorate from Utkal University in 1996.

He continued to give full evening recitals until his death in 2004. He earned huge acclaim as a dancer, teacher and *pakhawaj* player. He has established *Srjan* in Bhubaneswar for imparting training in Odissi dance. Today, his son, Ratikanta, who has developed into a good dancer and *pakhawaj* player, assists him in his work. Details of his life and his evolution as a *guru* has been documented in a book entitled "The making of a *Guru* – Kelucharan Mohapatra – his life and times" (Citaristi, 2001).

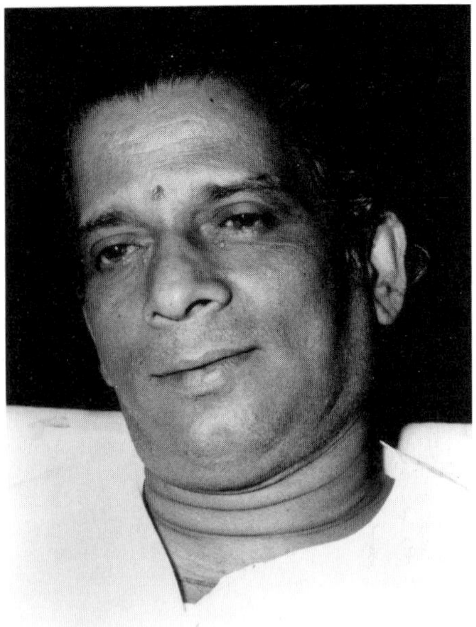

Guru Debaprasad Das, 1978 (courtesy: Central Sangeet Natak Akademi, New Delhi).

DEBAPRASAD DAS

Debaprasad Das, who passed away untimely at the age of 54 on 16th July 1986, was the youngest of the three *gurus*. His background was very different from the other *gurus*. He was born in 1932, in Keul Chabi Sua village in Jhankada, which is famous for the Sarala temple in Cuttack district. His father, Durga Charan Das, was a police inspector. His mother, Indramani Devi, died when he was only a year old. Debaprasad was exposed to music from his early childhood as his paternal grand-father, Bauribandhu Das, *gumastha* (accountant) by profession, was a good violin player and the music director of the Keul Natya troupe. He taught young Debaprasad the traditional music of Orissa – *chhanda, chaupadi, keshab koili, kanta koili, manobodh chautisa, abakasa*, etc. Later, he went to Puri to stay with his maternal uncle and there he attended school, but he showed least interest in studies and was drawn more to dance, drama, *jatra*, painting, etc. Often he used to sneak into the *Pathara akhada* and watch *Ram Leela* being staged in Janhimandia, Puri.

Occasional punishment did not cool his passion for music and dance. He started taking dance lessons secretly from the legendary *gotipua Nrityaguru* Mohan Charan Mohapatra of the *Pathara akhada*. With great difficulty he passed his minor (elementary school) examination and left for Ganjam district where his father was posted. Here, too, he neglected his studies to learn painting and terracota sculpture from Prahlad Patel. This led to discontent and frequent punishment at home. In 1944, he ran away from home and was employed as an actor in New theatres till 1949. As was the practice in those days, he took female roles in some plays. He became very popular as a comedian and subsequently he joined Annapurna theatre where he had a lot of scope, both as a dancer and a comedian. During this time, he had the opportunity to learn the rudiments of various classical and folk dances from Guru Kumar Dayal Sharan of Madras. In the early 50's, when a lot of eager students started learning dance and music, Debaprasad started teaching *gotipua* dance to young boys.

A turning point in his career came when he taught Odissi under the supervision of *Kabichandra* Kalicharan Patnaik for Priyambada's performance in the first Inter-University Youth Festival in Delhi, in 1954. Soon after this, Indrani Rehman, who had made quite a name for herself as a Bharatnatyam dancer, took training in Odissi from Debaprasad at the instance of Charles Fabri and the late Mayadhar Mansinha. For the next five years, Debaprasad trained Indrani and presented Odissi before National and International audiences. This was the period when he received wide recognition and honour. Students flocked to him. He joined Utkal Sangeet Mahavidyalaya in the early 60's as a lecturer in Odissi dance and continued to teach there till his untimely death. However, he was able to train a number of dancers including Vijaylaxmi Mohanty.

Debaprasad was the first to venture out of Orissa and gain exposure to other forms of classical dance. From this he drew some themes and movements which he used in his later choreography. However, in the final analysis, he was the most conservative of the three *gurus*. He was a stickler for the old Odissi with its "earthy" movements. He totally disapproved modern day Odissi costume – he never used stitched dresses. Thus, in his repertoire, one can see flashes of Odissi as it used to be in the 40's and 50's. His items are popular because of this very earthiness; they are the ones most performed in Orissa. His popular repertoire includes numbers like *astashambhu, thai-nata* (equivalent of *batu* and retaining the traditional from), *pallavis* in *ragas* like *kalyani, basanta, kalavati* and *mokshya* (again retaining the traditional form). His *abhinayas* are totally devoid of *sancharis*, adhering strictly to the *bhava* of the lyrics. He used Oriya lyrics more in his earlier compositions than the Sanskrit ones. His typical items like *Dasamahavidya* and *Nabarasa* became instant hits when he and his disciples presented them at the Angahar festival in Delhi, in 1985.

In many ways, Debaprasad's life was a sad one. Although he was a pioneer in the propagation and popularization of Odissi, national recognition came to him rather late in his career. He received the Orissa Sangeet Natak Akademi Award for dance in 1973, Central Sangeet Natak Akademi Award in 1977, and an award from World Development Corporation in 1983. He also received a senior fellowship from the Department of Culture, Government of India, for his research on "Dance as a ritual in Jagannath – *Seva* and *Akhanda Sampradaya*". He left a valuable manuscript, *Nrutyanusarani*, on the practical aspects of Odissi. There is no doubt that Debaprasad Das played a very critical role in the development and popularization of Odissi, deviating least from its traditional form.

REFERENCES

Citaristi, Ileana, 2001. *The Making of a Guru: Kelucharan Mohapatra, His Life and Times*, Manohar, New Delhi.

Mohanty-Hejmadi, Priyambada, 1990. "The Trinity of Odissi", *Sangeet Natak*, No. 96, pp. 3-18.

Patnaik, Kalicharan, (undated). *Odissi Dance* (technical consultants, *Singhari* Shyama Sunder Kar and Mahadev Rout), National Music Association, Cuttack.

Singh, Durllav Chandra, 1998. A *Satabdira Oriya Rangamancha and My Role*, Durllav Chandra Singh, Puri.

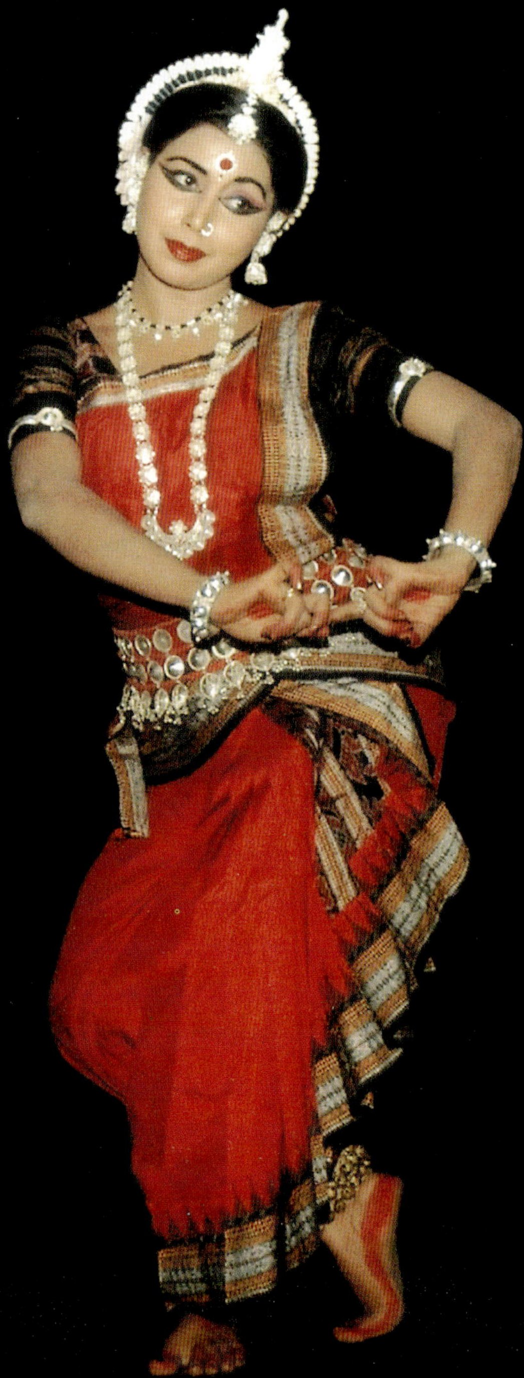

ODISSI MUSIC AND TEXTS

5

It has been rightly said that it is possible to have music without dance but it is impossible to have dance without music. In most of the types of classical dance in India, we have a specific type of music. For example, Carnatic style of music is used in Bharatnatyam and Kuchipudi dance forms, while Hindustani style of music is used for Kathak. The music used for Odissi dance is called Odissi music. This is the only classical dance where both the dance and music go by the same nomenclature, *i.e.*, Odissi.

Odissi music is a separate music system with distinctive features. The tradition of music was well established by the 12th century as the Sanskrit *astapadis* are unique compositions in which the immortal poet of Orissa, Jayadeva, has specified specific *ragas* and *talas* for each *astapadi*. The practice of documentation on palm leaves has meant a great loss of old manuscripts of dance and music in Orissa. However, many important manuscripts on dance and music, written between the 16th to 18th century, have survived the ravage of time.

Out of these, the most important ones are *Geeta Prakash* by Krushnadasa Badajena Mohapatra, *Natya Manorama* and *Sangitarnaba Chandrika* by Pandit Raghunath Rath, *Sangeeta Kalpalatika* by Kavi Shri Haladhara Mishra, *Sangeeta Narayana* by Kaviratna Purusottam Mishra, and *Abhinaya Darpana Prakasha* by Raja Jadusingh Mohapatra.

Sangeeta Kaumudi is considered to be the oldest text of music in Orissa. It is believed to be written in the 15th century and the name of the author still remains unknown. It has eight *padas* (chapters) devoted to Swaranirupana, Raganirupana, Talaswarupanirupana, Talanirupana, Bandhanirupana, Grahadinirupana, and Geetanirupana. The last chapter seems to be incomplete (Das, 1986).

Geeta Prakash is a treatise on the *geeta* and is exclusively devoted to vocal music. Panigrahi (1983) opines that the author Krishnadasa Badajena Mahapatra was an eminent poet, musician and musicologist of 16th century Orissa. *Geeta Prakash* consists of seven *ullasas* (chapters), namely Suddhageetanirnaya, Salanganirnaya, Kshudrageetanirnaya, Guṇnanirnaya, Raganirnaya, Swaranirnaya and Doshanirnaya. Thus, all the chapters relate to different aspects of *geeta*. It is important to mention that according to the eminent historian Mahapatra (1958), Krishnadasa Badajena Mahapatra is the "Mahapattra" in the court of Akbar, about whom Abul-i-Fazl writes:

> "Mahapattar", who was unrivalled in the arts of Indian poetry and the music, was sent along with him (Hasan Khan Khazanci). These two went together to Orissa to carry on negotiation about an alliance with Gajapati Mukunda Deva against the Nawab of Bengal in 1565 AD.

The book *Sangeetamuktabali*, written by Harichandan belonging to the royal family of Kanika, has been edited by Pandit Banambar Acharya (1955) who places the publication around 1590. The book is divided into four *grathanas* (chapters). The first *grathana* contains discussions on the different aspects of music, the second deals with *dhatu, matu, raga-raginis*, the third with *talas*, and the fourth mainly deals with *geeta* (vocal music), ending with a brief description of *badyalakshana* and *nrutya prakaranam*.

Sangeeta Kalpalatika, written by Shri Haladhar Mishra in the early part of the 17th century, deals with *geeta, vadya* and *nritya* and contains 18 chapters. Panigrahi (1984), who has edited the manuscript, is of the opinion that it was composed around 1635 AD. The treatise is the first of its kind written in Orissa according to Shri Panigrahi. The work is divided into 18 *stavakas* (chapters), seven of which are devoted to *geeta*, ten to *nritya* and one to *vadya*. The chapters have been explicitly named. The seven chapters on *geeta* are Shuddhageetanirupana, Chhayalaganirupana, Ksudrageetanirupana, Gananirupana, Dosanirupana, Raganirupana, Svaranirupana. The eighth chapter devoted to *vadya* is called Vadyanirupana The rest of the chapters are devoted to *Natya* consisting of Natyanirupana, Hastaknirupana, Shirovyaparanirupana, Dristinirupana, Bhruksepanirupana, Sthanakanirupana, Chareenirupana, Karanirupana, Kalasanirupana and Suddhapaddhatinirupana.

One of the most important text is *Sangeetarnaba Chandrika*. The author, Pandit Raghunath Rath, has dedicated the book to Raja Neelakantha of Kerala. Although it was assumed that Kerala refers to the modern day Kerala, based on the information given by the author himself in *Sangeetarnaba Chandrika*, Mishra (1983) has opined that the author actually refers to the small estate of Kerala in the east of Brahmani river which is now known as "Kalakala" of Cuttack district. Raja Neelakantha was very fond of music and Raghunath Rath was his "Sava Pandit". Pandit Raghunath wrote texts on music and dance. One was *Natya monorama* written around 1697 to 1698 and *Sangitarnaba Chandrika* written around 1689-90.

Sangitarnaba Chandrika (see Panigrahi, 1995) has five parts devoted to music, *raga*, *geeta*, *tala* and *vadya* and *nrutya*. The first part contains the origin and nature of music, the second part deals with *raga* and *raginis*, the third part relates to *geeta* (vocal music), the fourth part relates to *tala*, and finally the fifth part relates to *vadya* (instrumental music) and dance.

Natya Manorama (Rath, 1959) contains five *padas* (chapters), the first on music in general, the second on *ragas* and its *lakshanas*, the third on *talas*, the fourth on *geeta* (songs), and the last on *vadyas* (musical instruments) and dance.

Perhaps the most important document from the point of view of controversy is *Abhinaya Chandrika*, exclusively on *odra nrutya* written by Maheswara Mohapatra from the court of Sriman Naryanadeva of Khemundi Kingdom. The book has been published by the eminent scholar Pandit Sadasiva Ratha Sharma (1967) under the auspices of Raghunandan Library, Puri.

I am not competent enough to vouch for or against the authenticity of the manuscript. However, it contains surprising details of different aspects of dance which can be directly related to the modern day Odissi dance. The book starts with the *Ganapati bandana*, *"Namami Bighnarajamtam Kalpabrikshya talasthitam"*–a *sloka* frequently used for *Mangalacharan* in Odissi.

Although Shri Rath Sharma thinks that it was published in the 15th century, the eminent historian Kedarnath Mahapatra (1978), based on evidence from the reference quoted in it, opines that *Abhinaya Chandrika* was written in the first part of the 17th century during the time of Narayan Anangabhima Deva.

Apart from mentioning about the origin of *Udra nrutya* (Odissi *nrutya*) and its emphasis on expressional gestures (*bhaba*), it mentions about the different types of dance in Utkal (Orissa). According to the treatise, there were a variety of dance prevalent in Utkal which included *Jugma nrutya* (duet dance), dances during festivals which included folk themes on the *Ghotak* (performer dressed as a horse) or *Danaba* (performer dressed as a demon). It classifies *Danda nrutya* under *tandava*.

An interesting reference has been made to *Purusha nrutya* which the writer interprets as men dressed as girl dancers or *Gotipua nrutya*. According to the author, although *Gotipua nrutya* was popular it was of a lower status because the *gotipua* was not able to express his feelings through song and gestures in comparison to the girl dancers. But it was preferable to send *gotipuas* to entertain the Jabana (Muslim) kings because girl dancers will be ostracised in society for being touched by Muslim kings. Sometimes *Gotipua nrutya* was also held in the temples and in the palaces of kings.

Mahapatra (1978) opines further that due to the clear evidence of the existence of "Udra or Odissi dance" up to at least 12th century in Orissa, it is not fair to say that it originated from *Mahari* dance (ritual dance) at Jagannath temple.

Sangeeta Narayana, written by Kaviratna Purusottam Mishra (1966), is a better known musical text from Orissa. The book has been dedicated to Parlakhemundi Raja Jagannath Narayan Deva (1718-1769). It has four *parichhedas* (chapters) on *geeta nirnaya, badya nirnaya, natya nirnaya* and *bhasha nirnaya*. Thus, the third *parichheda* is important from dance point of view as it contains detailed discussions on *Dristi, Shira, Kara, Sthanaka, Karana, Bhusana*, and different types of dance, etc.

Raja Jadusingh Mahapatra of the then state Tigiria, compiled the treatise *Abhinaya Darpana Prakasha* in the first part of 19th century. It is an adaptation of "Abhinaya darpana" with much original contribution by the author. It is a very important treatise, exclusively devoted to dance. In addition to the descriptions of different types of dance, it has elaborate descriptions of different aspects in dance from *Sthanakas* to *Hasta binijoga*.

In addition, *Sangeeta Sara boli, Sangeeta Shastra, Sangeeta Sudhanidhi, Sangeeta Suravi, Sangeeta Ratna, Geeta Prakash Boli, Tala Nirnaya, Tala Nirupana, Tala Sarbasara* and *Tala Malika* are some of the other important but less known texts on music in Orissa (Das, 2000).

CHRONOLOGICAL ORDER OF TEXTS OF DANCE AND MUSIC IN ORISSA

Name	*Date*
Sangeeta Kaumudi	15th century
Geeta Prakash	1565
Sangeeta Muktabali	1590
Sangeeta Kalpalatika	1635
Sangeetarnaba Chandrika	1689-1690
Natya Manorama	1697-1698
Abhinaya Chandrika	17th century
Sangeeta Narayana	1718-1769
Abhinaya Darpana Prakasha	19th century.

In comparision to Hindustani and Carnatic style of singing, Odissi music has a very distinctive style. In a way, stylistically, it is somewhat in between the two styles being rendered in *andolita gamak*. In addition, *ahat, dhalu, kuṙala gamaks* are profusely used in Odissi music. The medieval *Ritiyuga* poets in Oriya literature have enriched Odissi music by recommending many *raga-raginis* and *talas* peculiar to Odissi music. To name a few, in Kalyan *anga* are *Chintakalyan, Purikalyan* and *Manjukalyanika*; in Kamodi *anga* are *Kedarkamodi, Shokakamodi, Kumbhakamodi, Odissikamodi, Sadhukamodi* and *Chandrikakamodi*; in Kedar *anga* are *Kalahansakedara, Shrikedara, Basantakedara* and *Mohanakedara*; in Gauda *anga* are *Malashrigauda, Kedaragauda* and *Salagagauda*; and in Baradi *anga* are *Panchamabaradi, Shoskabaradi*, etc. Similarly, the peculiar *talas* recommended are *Jati, Adtali, Nishari, Kuduka* and *Sarimana*.

Odissi music is rendered in different forms, namely *Odissi, Champu, Chhanda, Chautisha* and devotional (*Jananas, Bhajans*, etc). In addition, there are purely musical items without any lyrics like *Swaramalika, Lakshana Geeta* and *Pallavi*.

Odissi is divided into four types: *Dhrubapadanga, Raganga, Bhabanga* and *Natyanga* (Das, 1989). *Dhrubapanga* is rendered in *Dhrubapadanga* or *Dhrupad style. Malashri, Kuduka Geeta, Matha Geeta* and *Sariman Geeta* are rendered in this style. *Raganga* lyrics of *Ritijuga* poets are rendered in specific *raga* and *tala* with considerable elaboration in both. In *Bhabanga,* same lyrics may be used with limited elaboration for expression of the proper *bhava. Natyanga* is more perky and rendered in a light mode, which has been very popular for *gotipua* dance.

Champu means compositions with both *gadya* and *padya*. However, in Odissi music it has a different connotation. The lyrics, commonly known as *champu*, are written in the 34 *byanjana barna (ka to khsya)* with specified *ragas.* The peculiarity is that each line of the lyric begins with the same alphabet and is referred to accordingly. For example, the popular *Bhangi chahan* is referred to as *Bha Champu*. They belong to the *Manushi matruka kshudra geeta* style. Each *champu* is sung in specific *raga* and *tala.*

Chhanda derives its name from the *chhanda, bani* or *brutta*. Like in Sanskrit, there are specific *brutas* in Oriya literature. Poets have specified *chhandas* for each composition. This tradition continues till today. Some of the more popular *chhandas* or *brutas* are *Gadamalia, Chakrakeli, Chokhi, Munibarabani, Koili, Kalasa, Rasakulya* and *Ashadhashukla*, etc. The *chhanda* style of singing does not contain varieties of *antaras* but is rendered in the same *swara* in a specific *tala*, creating moods pertaining to the lyrics. It is said that whether one understands the language or not, *chhanda* touches the soul!

Chautisha literally means the 34 alphabets. Each song has 34 sections starting with *ka* and ending with *kshya*. They are lengthy and are rendered in *chhanda* style without any ornamentation.

Devotional songs include *jananas* and *bhajans*. They are distinct, both from composition and rendering points of view. *Jananas* are appeals to the Lord and *bhajans* are in praise of the Lord. *Jananas*, therefore, have a strong desperate and, at times, accusing mood while *bhajans* are more submissive. It is a peculiarity that as mentioned in the relevant chapter, in the famous *Sarpa janana Kabisurya*, Baladeva Rath has literally rebuked Lord Jagannath as the biggest and meanest serpent of all! However, in both the dominant *bhaha* is *bhakti*. Some of the *bhajans* are rendered by the singing minstrels like *Nathas* and *Jogis* and take the name of the accompanying instruments like *kendara geeta* or *khanjani bhajan*, respectively.

Coming to the relation of Odissi music to Odissi dance, it has been said that the pleasant appealing quality of Odissi music has contributed significantly to the popularisation of Odissi dance. In general narrative *slokas* in praise of gods and goddesses are now rendered in specific *ragas* and *talas*. However, for *bhumipranam* and the final piece, specific *bols* are used in which *mardala* and *gini* are used along with the oral chanting of *ukutas.* Unfortunately, there is a tendency to match the rhythm with music these days which interferes with the mood of the piece. In *Batu* or *Sthayi* or *Thai*, which is pure dance, the syllables are rendered in a typical style. *Pallavi* is pure music in which considerable variations in both *tala* and *laya* are explored. This is the piece which has undergone the most expansion as initially the *pallavis* were short and used to flow into *abhinaya* in the same *raga* without any break and used to be called *Sabhinayapallavi.* However, with the two being distinct units, now the *raga* of the *pallavi* is usually different from that of *abhinaya.* The *pallavi* used to be simplistic, both from music and dance point of view, but now has become very ornate. *Pallavis* were known as *Tarijhams* as the *bani* is mainly *tarijham-ritajhina*, etc. However, later some have been composed with only *Sa Re Ga Ma*, etc. *Pallavis* are named after the *raga* in which they are composed but are mainly based on the tunes of traditional songs. The following is a list of *pallavis* and the tune of the song they are based upon.

Kalyan-Dekhiba para asare
Basant-Mana na kara more
Bilahari-Ajamu dekhili ghanashyamaku
Aravi-Ajashri gosthachandrama
Saveri-Nabaghanakalia kirangechanhila lo chaila
Shankarabharana-Chahanre nidhibara kalakushalaku

For *abhinaya, Odissi, chhanda, champu* and *bhakti geeta* are used. In addition, *astapadis* from *Gita Govinda* are extremely popular for *abhinaya*. It is said that the Odissi medium is extremely suitable for *astapadis. Mokshya* is the only piece in which music is not used. It is purely based on variations of *tala*. Presently, narrative *slokas* are used at the end sometimes.

REFERENCES

Acharya, Banamber, 1955. *Sangeetamuktabali*, Utkal University, Bhubaneswar.

Das, Ramahari, 1986. "Odissi Sangeeta Parampara Keteka Sangeetakara O' Sangeetakruti" (in Oriya), *Hansadwani*, Utkal Sangeet Mahavidyalayas, Bhubaneswar.

——. 1989. *Sangeeta Samgnya* (in Oriya), Kaishiki Prakashani, Bhubaneswar.

——. 2000. "Uchhanga Sangeeta" (in Oriya), *Odisha* (edited by Basant Das), Anusandhana Publication, Bhubaneswar.

Mahapatra, Krishnadas Badajena, 1983. *Geeta Prakash* (edited by Sri Nilamadhab Panigrahi), Orissa Sangeet Natak Akademi, Bhubaneswar.

Mahapatra, K.N., 1958. "Two Unknown Sanskrit Poets of Orissa", *The Orissa Historical Research Journal*, VII (II), pp. 73-82.

Mahapatra, Kedarnath, 1978. "Abhinaya Chandrika" barnita Udra Nrutya "Odissi nrutya" (in Oriya), *Orissi Nrutya Alochana*, Orissa Sangeet Natak Academy, Bhubaneswar, pp. 33-49.

Mahapatra, Maheswara, 1967. *Abhinava Chandrika* (annotated by Pandit Sadasiv Ratha Sharma), Raghunandan Library, Puri.

Mishra, Haladhara, 1984. *Sangeet Kalpalatika* (edited by Nilamadhab Panigrahi), Orissa Sangeet Natak Akademi, Bhubaneswar.

Mishra, Kaviratna Purosottam, 1966. *Sangeeta Narayana*, Orissa Sangeet Natak Akademi, Bhubaneswar.

Mishra, Nilamani, 1983. "Utkaliya Sangeeta Shastra and Shastrakara" in *Rangabhumi*. Orissa Sangeet Natak Akademy, Bhubaneswar, pp. 62-77.

Nilakantha, 1995. *Sangeetarnava Chandrika* (edited by Nilamadhab Panigrahi), Orissa Sangeet Natak Akademi, Bhubaneswar.

Panda, Bhagaban, 1984. "Sangeetarnaba Chandrika: Eka Adhyayana", *Rangabhumi*. Orissa Sangeet Natak Akademi, Bhubaneswar, pp. 1-15.

Panigrahi, Nilamadhab (ed.), 1995. *Abhinaya Darpana Prakash*, Culture Directorate, Govt. of Orissa.

Rath, Raghunath, 1959. *Natya Manorama*, Orissa Sahitya Akademi, Bhubaneswar.

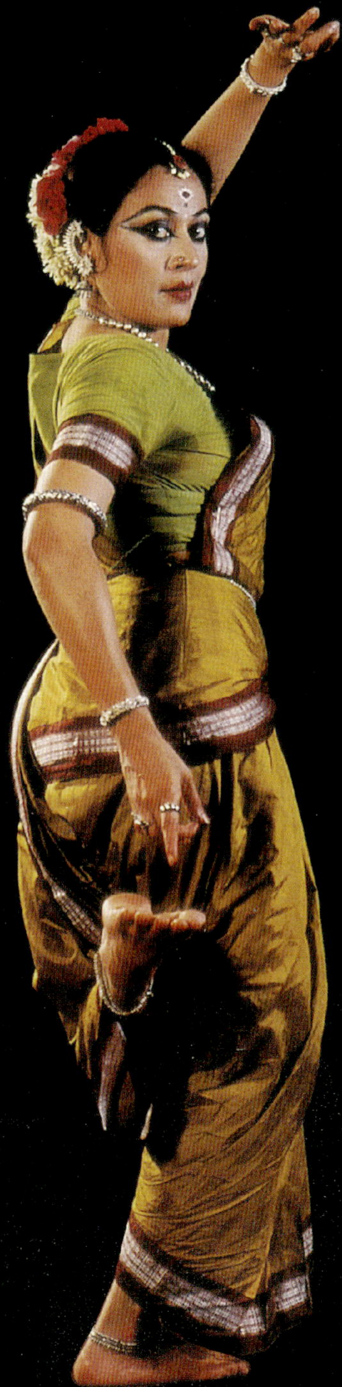

APPENDICES

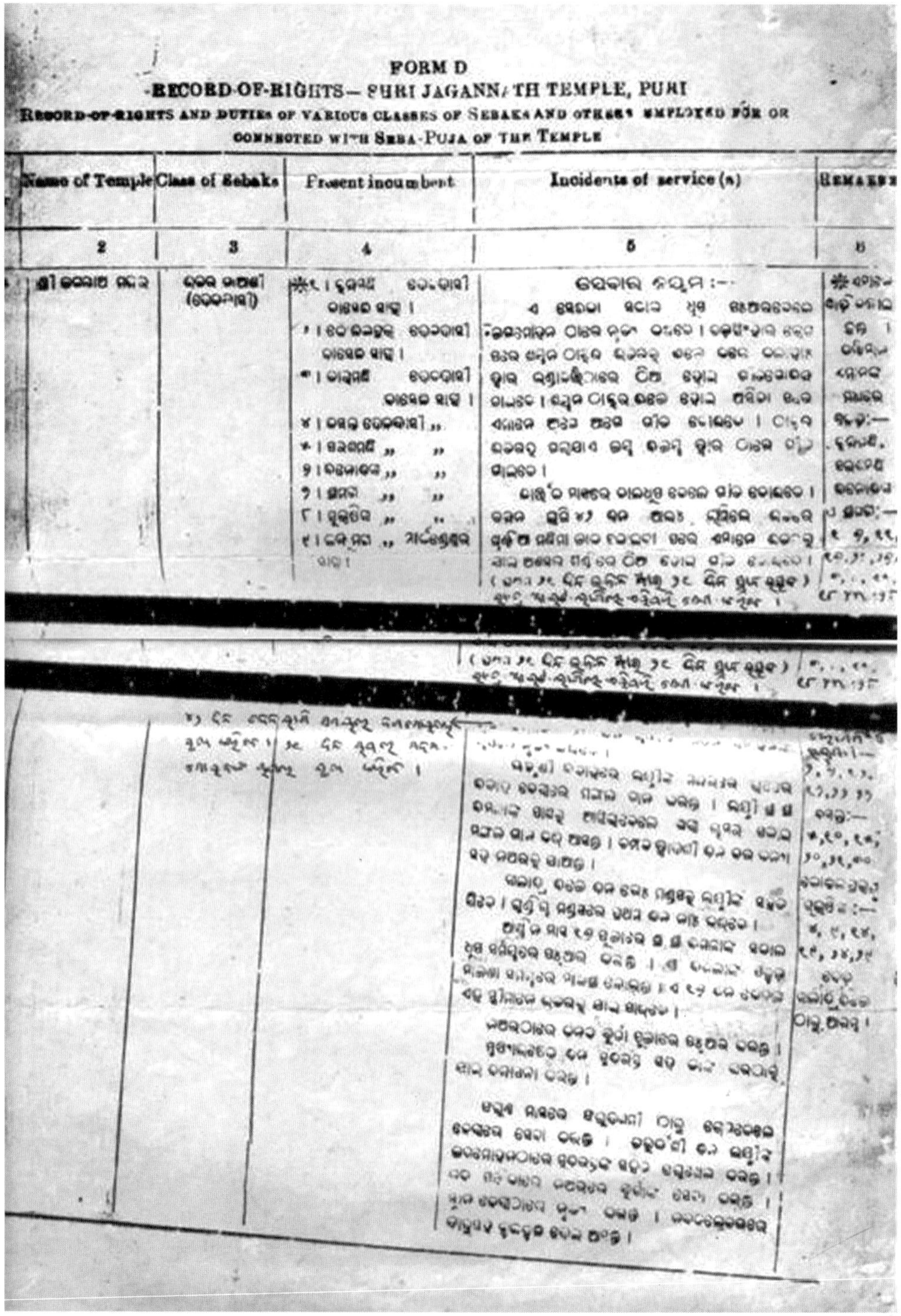

FORM D

RECORD-OF-RIGHTS— PURI JAGANNATH TEMPLE, PURI

RECORD-OF-RIGHTS AND DUTIES OF VARIOUS CLASSES OF SEBAKS AND OTHERS EMPLOYED FOR OR CONNECTED WITH SEBA-PUJA OF THE TEMPLE

Name of Temple	Class of Sebaks	Present incumbent	Incidents of service (a)	Remarks
2	3	4	5	6
[illegible]	[illegible]	[illegible]	[illegible]	[illegible]

Appendix 1. Record of Rights of Jagannath Temple, 1952

Part 1.

2	3	4	5	6
			[illegible]	[illegible]

L. PANDA
Special Officer
Under the Puri
Shri Jagannath Temple
Administration Act (Orissa
Act. 14 of 1952)

...Press, Cuttack

(a) Here record all particulars required in rule 8.

Part 2.

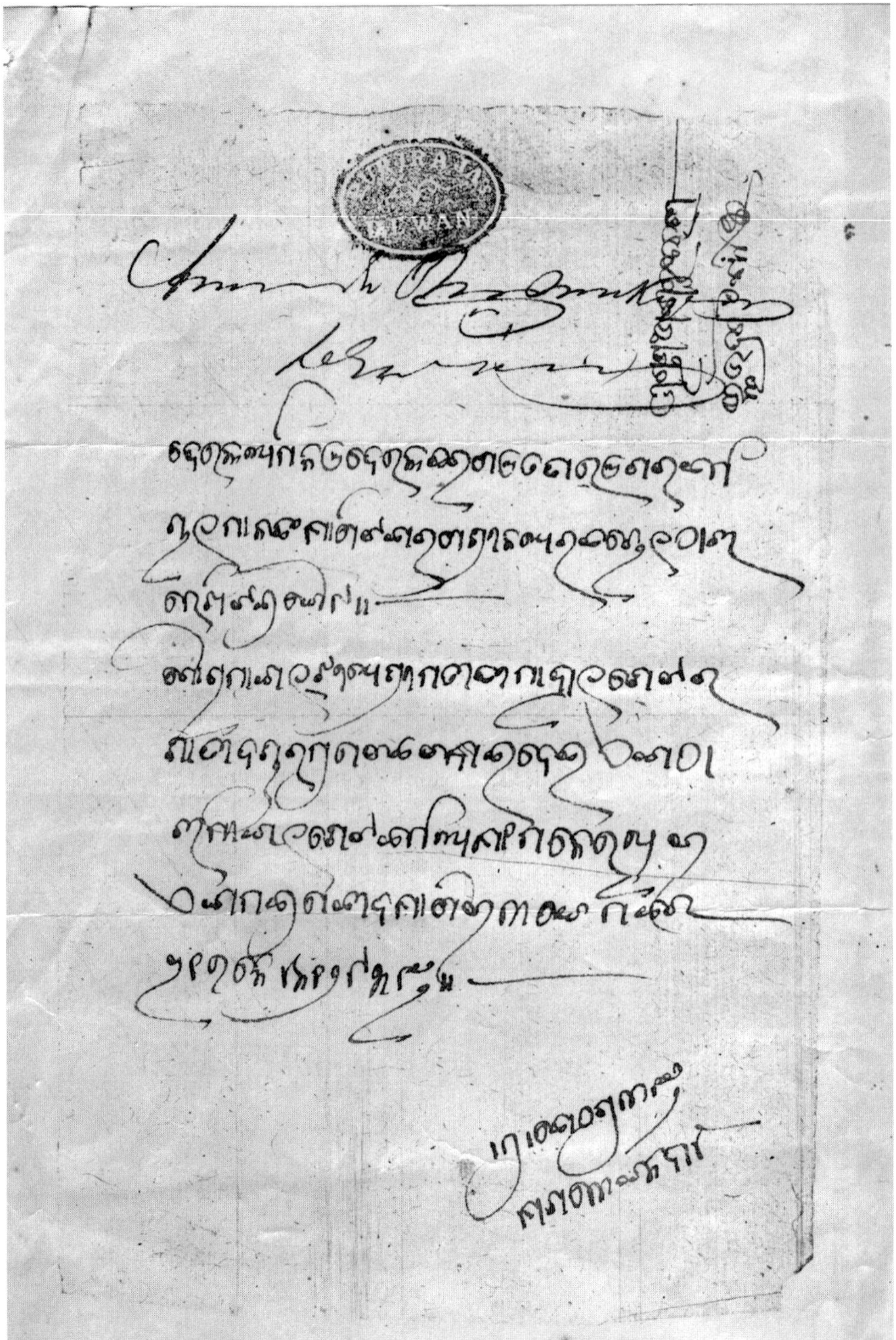

Appendix 2. Chhamu Chitau from Puri Raja Diwan issued in 1886 AD *for recruitment of Gauri Mahari's daughter Shrimati into Mahari seva.*

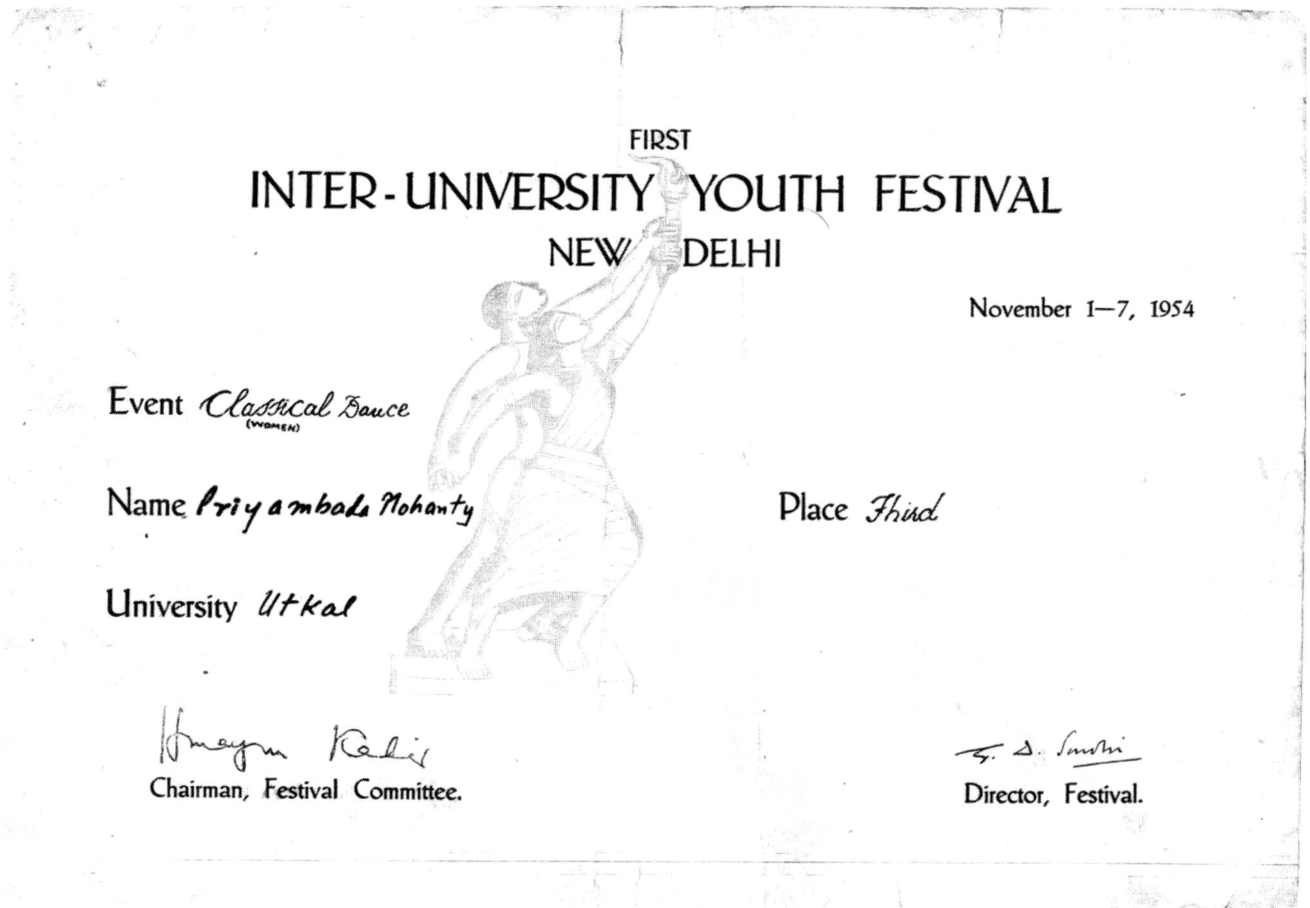
FIRST
INTER-UNIVERSITY YOUTH FESTIVAL
NEW DELHI

November 1—7, 1954

Event Classical Dance (WOMEN)

Name Priyambada Mohanty　　Place Third

University Utkal

Humayun Kabir
Chairman, Festival Committee.

G. D. Sondhi
Director, Festival.

Appendix 3. Certificate of Priyambada from First Inter-University Youth Festival 1954 signed by the then Education Minister Honourable Humayun Kabir (note that only Classical Dance is mentioned, the style is missing).

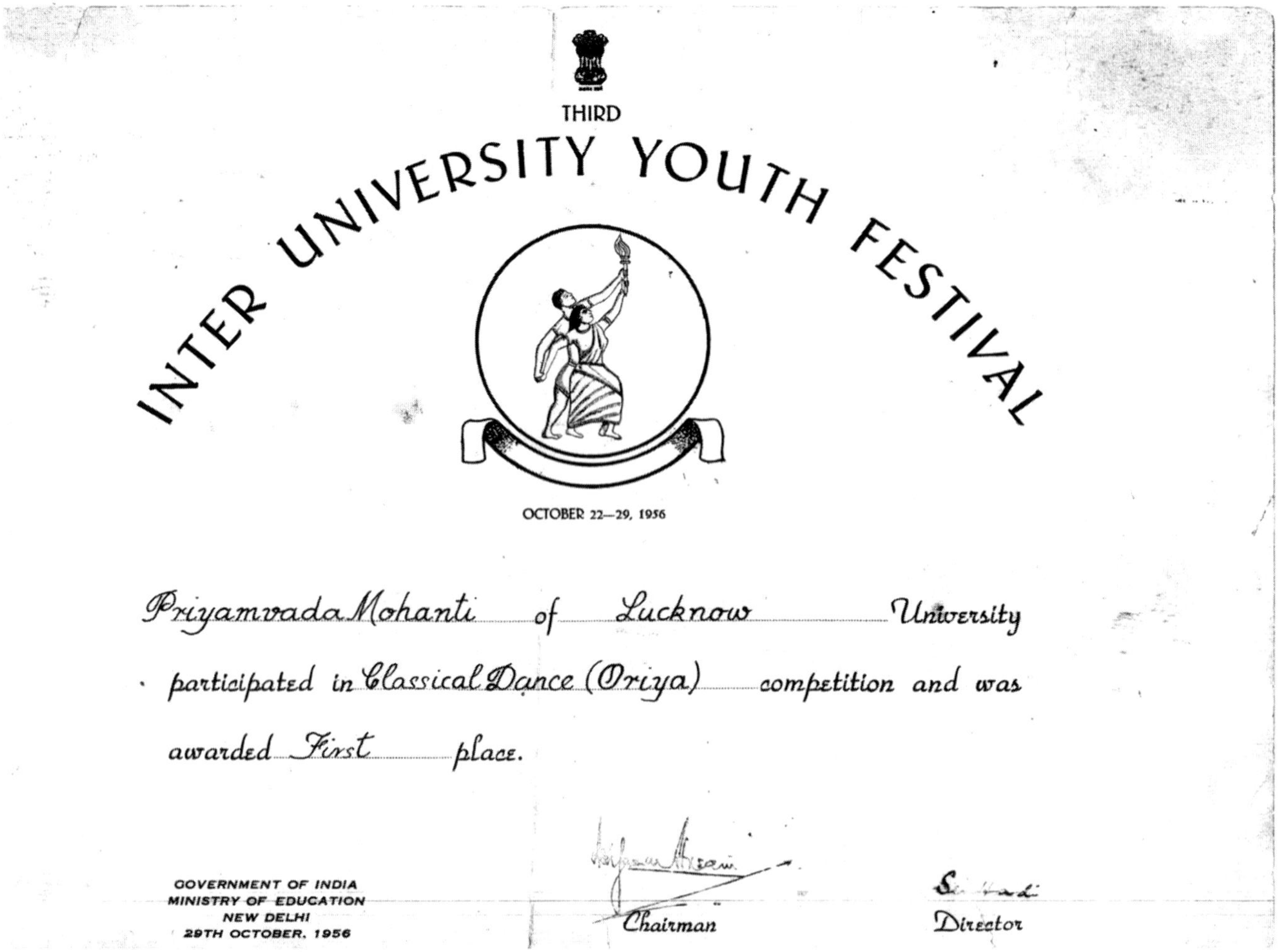
THIRD

INTER UNIVERSITY YOUTH FESTIVAL

OCTOBER 22—29, 1956

Priyamvada Mohanti of Lucknow University participated in Classical Dance (Oriya) competition and was awarded First place.

GOVERNMENT OF INDIA
MINISTRY OF EDUCATION
NEW DELHI
29TH OCTOBER, 1956

Chairman

Director

Appendix 4. Certificate of Priyambada from Third Inter-University Youth Festival 1956 (note that the style of classical dance is mentioned as Oriya).

THE LITTLE THEATRE GROUP

PRESENTS

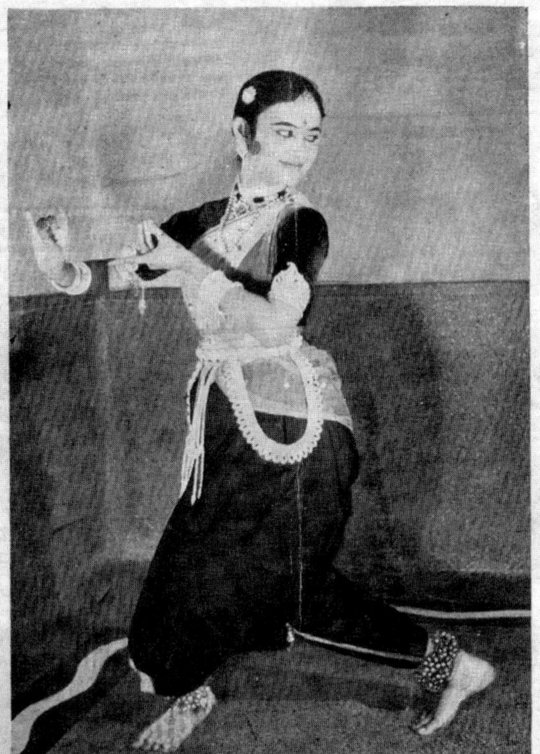

Priyambada Mohanty

October 14, 15 1961 at 6-30 P.M. — SAPRU HOUSE

Appendix 5 . Cover of The Little Theatre Group, New Delhi. Souvenir presenting the full evening programme in Odissi.

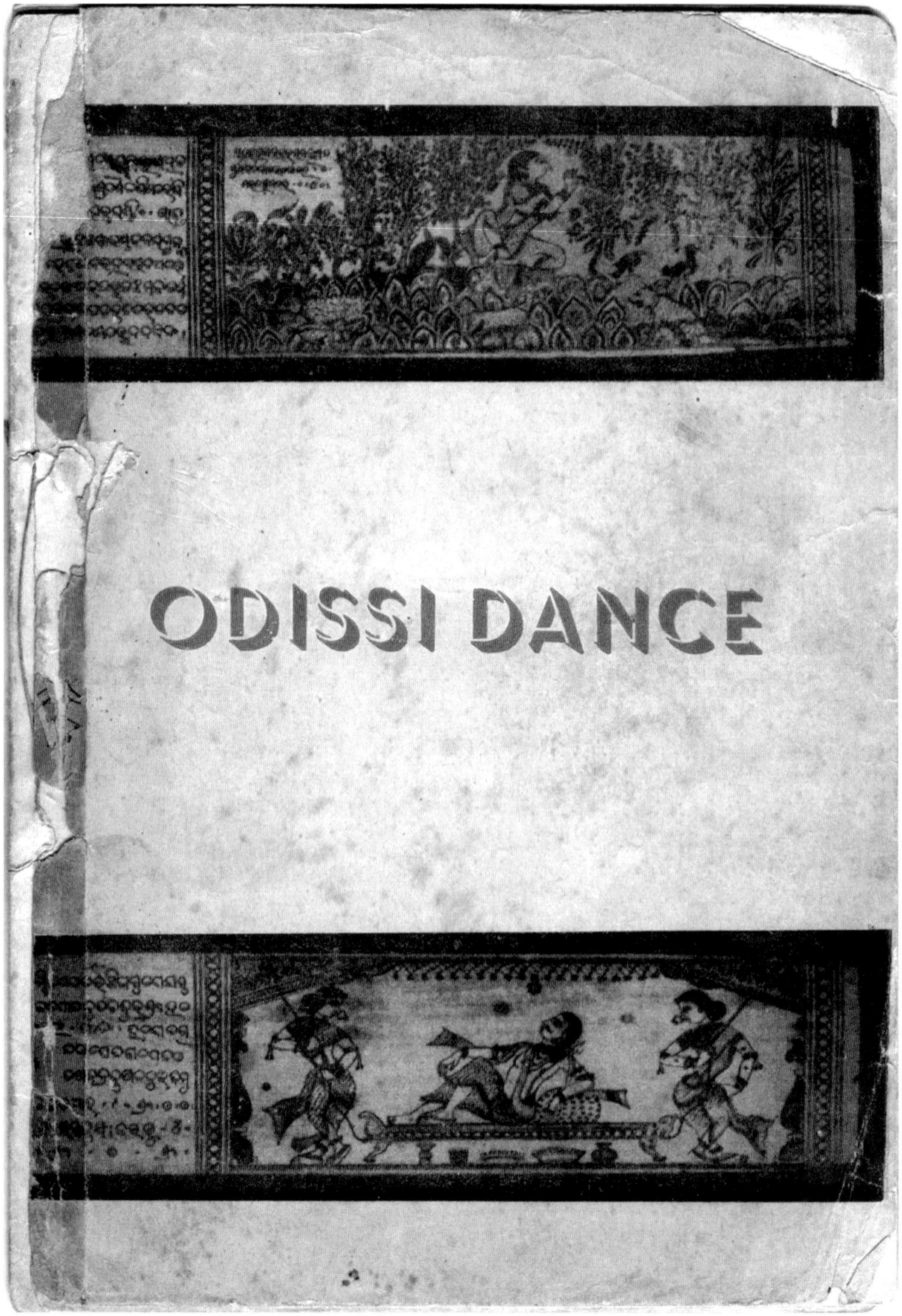

Appendix 6. Cover of the first book on Odissi Dance by Kavichandra Kalicharan Patnaik published by Utkal Nrutya Natyakala Parishad (Orissa Sangeet Natak Akademi at present) in 1954.

Glossary

Abhinaya: gestures to the lyrics of a song with the hands and facial expression

Ahia: the ladies who will never be a widow, for example being married to Lord Jagannath, the mahari enjoys a life-long ahia status

Akhada: gymnasium

Akhadagharas: gymnasium complex

Akshay Trutiya: an auspicious day coinciding with the 3rd day in the fullmoon phase of the lunar cycle in the month of Baishakh

Alasakanyas: beautiful young girls in sculpuresque poses used as charms in Orissa temples

Andolita gamak: characteristic wavy melodic movement of voice in Odissi music

Angabhangi: movement of different parts of the body

Apartiani: a child born after the death of a sibling

Ashikhita: illiterate

Badasinghara Vesha: ceremonial decoration of Lord Jagannath in the evening

Badasinghara: see *Badasinghara Vesha*
Bahuda: return
Bala dhupa: food offered to the deities in the morning
Bani: rhythmic syllables chanted while playing the *mardal/pakhwaj*
Bauddha Gana O' Doha: the first musically oriented poems of Orissa written by *Bauddha bhikshus*
Bedhas: the compound surrounding the temples
Bengapatia: an typical waist ornament made in silver with pieces strung in several rows with the pieces in the bottom row resembling the mouth of frog (Benga-frog; Patia-mouth)
Bhaba: synonym for *bhava*
Bhanati: prayer
Bhangi: posture
Bhava: expression
Bhumipranam: the tripartite salutation in the beginning of Odissi dance where a dancer pays her obeisance to the mother Earth (*Bhumi*), musicians and the audience
Brindabati: a typical feature in Oriya household representing the goddess in the form of a *Tulasi* plant on a pedestral
Brutas: typical patterns of lyrics in Orissa
Carnatic Music: music from south India
Chaitanya Charitamruta: a Bengali document on the life of the medieval saint *Shri Chaitanya* by Krushnadas Goswami, contains some important information on the music and dance in the medieval period in Orissa
Chamara Seva: the ritual of fanning with the flying whisk (*chamara*)
Chandana Jatra: the 21-day festival starting from akshay trutiya in the month of *Jyestha* during which the deities are taken for boat rides in the Narendra tank
Chandana Lagi: the process of application of sandalwood paste
Charchika: the one who decorates with sandalwood paste (*chandana*)
Charitamruta: synonymous with *Chaitanya Charitamruta*
Chauka: a characteristic posture in Odissi dance where the dancer creates four right angles at the shoulder, elbow, thigh and knee
Chaupadi: poems with four stanzas
Chautisa: lyrics like chhanda containing 34 stanzas
Chhamu-Chitau: official correspondence from Puri Raja

Chhanda: style of singing rendered in the same tune in specific brutas creating specific moods appropriate to the lyrics

Dakhsini: literally means from south but here it means the attire in south Indian style

Devadasi: maidens dedicated to Gods for specific rituals

Dewan: minister

Dhupa: meal, in Jagannath temple there are several offerings of meals during the different times during the day and they are identified by suffix. For example a morning meal is *sakala dhupa* etc.

Gamaks: tonal movements in music

Garuda Sthamba: the stone pillar with *Garuda* sitting atop in the dance hall of Jagannath temple since Lord Jagannath is an incarnation of Vishnu, *Garuda* finds a place in the temple

Garuda: the celestial bird, the carrier of Lord Vishnu

Gita Govinda: the book of poems written in Sanskrit by Shri Jayadeva in 12th century AD

Gini: small cymbals

Gotipua: boys of tender age trained in the art of dancing and singing

Guru Parampara: traditional imparting of training from generation to generation under the direct supervision of experts (*gurus*)

Guru: traditional revered teachers

Hasta binijoga: the rules governing the use of hands in classical dance. There are 24 *asamjukta hasta* (single hand) and 36 *samjukta hasta* (both hands) specified for the purpose.

Hastabhinaya: hand gestures in Indian classical dance used to depict the meaning of lyrics

Jabana: muslim

Jagamohana: the hall in front of the main temple (*Bimana*) in *Kalingan* architecture

Jananas: devotionational lyrics in the form of appeals to Gods and Goddesses

Jayadeva: the writer of *Gita Govinda* from Orissa

Jayantika: the organization of gurus, experts and dancers formed in late 1950's under the leadership of Shri Dhirendranath Patnaik to standardize the repertoire of Odissi dance

Jhoolan Jatra: the festival during the month of *Shravana* when the *gotipuas* perform in different maths (religious centres)

Jogis: singing ministrels

Kalghata Dwara: the last door leading to the sanctum sanctorum

Kanchala: the traditional blouse used by *maharis* during the rituals

Kendarageeta: specific songs used with the accompanying musical string instrument (*kendara*)

Khajanigeeta: specific songs used with the accompanying musical instrument (*khajani*)

Laya: tempo of music

Madeli: the one who plays the drum (*mardal*), a hereditary class attached to the Jagannath temple

Mahari: *devadasis* of Jagannath temple

Maluni: a lady supplying flowers

Manchapravesha: a ceremonial entry of a dancer to stage

Mandir: temple

Mangalacharan: the first item in Odissi repertoire which is used as invocation

Mardala: the accompanying drum used for Odissi dance, synonymous with *pakhawaj*

Mina Nahaka: over all in-charge for the ritual in the temple for the *maharis*.

Mokshya: the last item in Odissi repertoire

Mudra: hand gesture

Murdanga: a clay drum

Natamandira: dance hall used for dance, drama, music and other cultural activities, usually in the front portion of the temple

Natyacharya: expert in dance, drama and music

Natyashastra: the oldest treatise on dance, drama and music of India written by sage Bharata

Nijoga: duty, it is believed that at one time there were 36 types of duties (*chatisnijoga*) in the Jagannath temple

Nipa: synonym for *Kadamba* tree–frequently used by different poets as a favourite of Lord *Krishna*

Nritya: synonymous with *nrutya*

Nrityaguru: the dance teacher

Odissi: pertaining to Orissa state, dance is Odissi dance and music is known as Odissi music etc.

Oriya *lokanatya*: popular theatre in Oriya language

Pahada: closing

Pakhawaj: synonym for *mardala*

Pallavi: an item of pure dance in Odissi dance where the dancer elaborates on the musical variations

Pan: betel leaf, used for ceremonies and also eaten with several ingradients

Parikrama: the ceremonial walk around the temple

Puja: ritualistic offerings to gods and goddesses

Pujaka: priest

Raga Lakshanas: characteristic feature of *ragas*

Rama Leela: opera based on the theme of Lord Rama

Rasa Leela: opera based on Radha Krishna theme

Rathajatra: the 9-day car festival starting on the 2nd day of the full moon phase of the lunar cycle in the month of *Ashadha* when Lord Jagannath alongwith his elder Balabhadra and sister Subhadra come out of the temple and go to visit their their aunt Gundicha Devi

Ratnabedi: the pedestal of Lord Jagannath, elder brother Balabhadra and sister Subhadra inside the *sanctum sanctorum*

Record of Rights: the manual of Jagannath temple with the roster for different duties

Ritijuga: a particular literary period from the time of Bhanja to Gopalakrushna in medieval age

Sakala dhupa: morning meal

Sambhranta: aristocratic

Saribandha: ceremonial recruitment to different rituals in the Jagannath temple in which a piece of cloth is tied on the head of the initiated (here the cloth represents the *saree*–the traditional attire of women in Orissa)

Singhari: the person who decorates the deities in the Jagannath temple in the evening

Suanga: comedy

Tala: metrical pattern of tempo in music in different *matras* (units), there are nine such *talas* in Odissi music

Tarijham: synonymous with *pallavi* where a dancer elaborates on musical patterns by pure dance (the nomenclature is from the peculiar syllables–*tari, jham, jhenu* etc, used in the music)

Ukutas: rhythmic syllables

Ustads: experts in music

Vedi: platform or pedestal. for the images of gods and goddesses

Vidwan: expert

Vighnaraja: Lord Ganesh
Vihara: recluse
Vimana: the parapet on the temples
Zamindar: landlords appointed during the British rule
Zari: trimmings with threads of silver and gold

Index